Awaken
to
Agelessness

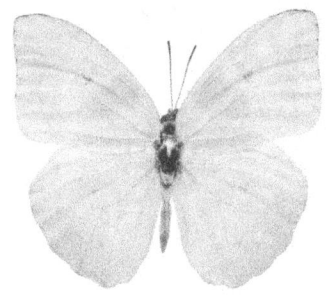

Also by Joy McMahon

Ageless At 75

Awaken to Agelessness

Joy McMahon

Table of Contents

Preface

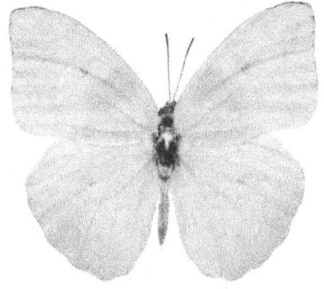

Preface

My personal journey into Agelessness began in 2008, while I was staying in Hawaii for six weeks. I experienced a sudden and profound realization while walking on the beach one day, on how to reverse my biological clock, and to slow down my aging process! My first book was published later that year, and the title was "Ageless at 75." It is now out of print. By popular demand while nearing 82, I am offering the revised version of this book which includes more updated information.

You will learn how to tap into your "Inner Power" (which is using the higher energy of consciousness) that will help you to become ageless and filled with vitality. You will learn how to regenerate yourself at the cellular level. You will discover how your biological clock works, and how you can reset it to slow down the aging process. The results will be solely up to you, as it involves your belief about yourself, and how well you apply the inner and outer work that needs to be done for manifesting agelessness. What we personally believe and put into practice inwardly is what we will manifest outwardly. All facets for reaching agelessness can be found in this book from the interior design of self, to the outer design!

Harvard University and other Universities have conducted many studies on the power of the mind in action with MRI Scans. They have found that using the power of the focused mind through meditation practice, showed positive changes in the entire brain function. Being ageless, means you must have a vital brain/mind along with a healthy and strong body.

How My Personal Journey Began:

My interest in health and vitality began way back in the 1970's when I visited a doctor who practiced the alternative healing art of Acupressure, in Santa Barbara California. I needed a correction for a physical condition, and I wanted to see what this natural therapy would do for me. The positive results of the therapy made me a believer and a client.

From then on, my interest in Acupressure and other alternative healing methods peaked, and led me into my own career in natural healing. I studied Acupressure in California, and later became the first certified Acupressure therapist in the state of Washington, in early 1980.

I was such an oddity and pioneer in alternative health practices, that our local newspaper "The Spokesman Review" published a full page story about my work (with colored photos), and one of our local TV stations followed, by airing my work as a "prime time" special, that was viewed as far as Canada. Suddenly, I had a large following of clients!

My career developed into teaching and speaking in the year of 1984, which included speaking in hospitals, schools, and for conventions and organizations. My talks were about how to live a healthy life, managing stress, and about healing through Acupressure, and other valid healing modalities.

I created a manual on Acupressure Facelift, and taught this method in our local community college, along with another course on First Aid Acupressure. Again, the local newspaper found me, and published another full page (with colored photos) about my work with Acupressure for natural facial rejuvenation. Learning how to be ageless began to fascinate me even then, as well as capturing the interest of the public.

In the 1990's I took courses in Yoga and Stress Management and became certified in both. I opened one of the first Yoga studios in Spokane, Washington, shortly after I completed my training. At the same time, I became increasingly aware that our thoughts had the power to make a positive difference in the health and rejuvenation of our physical body! I still continue to teach Yoga to seniors up to ninety years, and to baby boomers.

One interest continued to segue into another. In the year of 1993 I became concerned about the then, newly revealed field of bio-genetically engineered food. I connected with the Union of Concerned Scientists, based in Washington D.C. I began to communicate with them, and they sent me a wealth of information. With all of this documented information in hand, I personally visited all the major grocery stores in Spokane, with my concerns over Bovine Growth Hormones being added to our milk supply, and genetically altered food, that would soon be marketed to the public. It fell on deaf ears!

Later, I connected with Jeremy Rifkin who was the President of the Washington D.C. based foundation for Economic Trends, and author of books that questioned the ethics of the new bio-genetic engineered technologies, especially related to our food, which of course involved the farm and dairy communities.

To bring awareness to the public, I invited Mr. Rifkin to speak at the Pacific Northwest Farm Forum. It was such a controversial subject that armed security guards stood by. Many TV and news reporters followed me around, wanting information from the woman who had caused such a stir, by inviting Rifkin to speak! Being in the news again, many Washington state parents called me with concerns about the Bovine Growth hormones being added to milk.

Because, of our altered food by high technology, and all of the additives and heavy pesticides used in farming, this has caused me to choose organic food. I also stay away from all milk products that contain the added hormones and are not from grass fed cows.

Still getting the word out about health in 2005, I was a regular columnist for the periodical, "Dimensions" that was published in Virginia Beach, Virginia. My articles were about living a healthy lifestyle, and offering ideas for rejuvenation. I also wrote articles about "positive thinking" for the Northwest Woman magazine, and the Family magazine, both published in Spokane.

Since then, I have focused my full attention and intention on Agelessness, teaching Yoga classes with meditation, and offering workshops and speaking engagements about Stress Management and Agelessness, and publishing this book.

My blessings to you.

Introduction

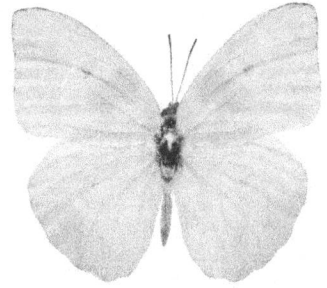

The Journey Into Agelessness

You might be questioning what determines Agelessness? Being agelessness is a person where age cannot be defined accurately due to appearance. Agelessness is also attributed to individuals whose physical and mental characteristics appear young for their biological age.

Having facial cosmetic surgery or body contour surgery, or adding Botox and other fillers and treatments to the face is not true agelessness. This is only a mask. True agelessness is created by "inner design" and "outer design" naturally, which promotes youthfulness. True agelessness is an art, and you are the artist. So, learn to make "Timeless Art" by using the information offered in this book!

When I give workshops I ask the following question. "Do you really believe that you have a powerful mind, one that is so powerful it can change your life for the better, and even stimulate youth in your cells?" Usually there is a resounding YES, because more and more people are waking up to the fact that our mind-set actually creates what we are! The power of the mind is being proven everyday by advanced science, and by many ordinary people, which includes me!

Personally, I have discovered the KEYS to age reversal, and how to slow down the aging process by programming a new inner design, that remains active in my consciousness, and reflects in my cells. Continuing on since 2008, I have accomplished reversing my age biologically. At eighty-two years in 2015, most people think I am at least ten years younger, and that is not the "old stereotype" of someone in the age bracket in their early seventies!

For some people, old age begins in their fifties or sooner, because they THINK they are getting old. They reinforce old age every time they think or say, "I am getting older." Then, they start acting like they are thinking, and their consciousness and body responds to their enforced belief.

I have always known that in order to have a sense of wellness and youthful vitality, I needed to pay attention to good health habits, and the practice of positive and affirmative mental habits. I have not always been totally consistent in my awareness of self-care but, for the majority of my adult years I have taken good care of myself. I have never bought into the "old age myth," and this has had a positive impact on all levels of my being.

Throughout my journey of life, I have learned that when I think positive thoughts, and when I let go of my perceptions about how things should be unfolding, I feel relaxed and stress free. My body then assumes a state of harmony. When I am relaxed that means I am in a trusting state of consciousness, and I know that all is well. When I feel all is well, and is as it should be, I am in a state of wellness or wholeness, and aging cannot make its' impact upon me. My lesson has been that there is always a reason for things to unfold as they are, because Spirit has a better plan for me than my ego has!

There are times when I feel worried, confused, fearful, and stressed like anyone else as life is not always easy! The good thing is, I usually lift myself out of these states of mind quickly because I am an aware person, and strive to live a conscious and positive life. When I completely let go of resistance and allow the plan of Spirit to take place, I flow naturally once again into timelessness. In timelessness, I am not rushed or worried because I am centered in the NOW.

In timelessness my biological clock slows down. Time cannot register anywhere in my consciousness when I am centered in the moment of relaxed awareness. My experience of time becomes subjective.

I also notice that I am in a state of timelessness when I am creating a work of art. I love to paint and to write, and **in my inner space of creativity, there is no time**. My biological clock slows way down in the act of creativity! In this state, I am ageless or timeless. The more I stay focused in the moment of now, the idea of time cannot invade my consciousness! NOW is all there is in reality.

~~~

In February of 2008, Spirit had a great awakening planed for me when I spent six long magical weeks in Hawaii. In this beautiful place it was easy for me to be in the "now" most of the time, especially when I was walking alone in Paradise!

While I was there, my consciousness shifted into a higher level of understanding about cellular renewal. I began to receive information on how to live an ageless life by standing in my spiritual power and tuning into my DNA, so that my cells would respond, and come into perfect alignment. This information was fed to my conscious mind through Spirit. I immediately put this understanding into practice!

In a short time, I began to feel and look younger. My thought patterns became very focused on my intention. I was on a mission for self renewal! I not only began to experience regeneration at a cellular level, but spiritually as well.

During my stay on the beautiful island of Oahu, I walked for miles every day. While walking, I received more and more regenerative ideas. This is when I began to actually breathe in the information for reversing the aging process into my body's cells.

Upon returning to Spokane, I have continued to work on myself for rejuvenation. It is my desire to pass this valuable information along to my readers, so that you, too, can create a healthy, ageless life!

Before beginning this incredible journey for self renewal, you truly must be ready to make some major changes in your thought patterns, as well as how you treat your body. In fact, you must be open to making some major changes in your entire lifestyle! Remember, it is YOU that must do the work by tapping into your innate "magic" for youth and rejuvenation. There is no product or magic potion for real youth you are the magic-maker!

Step 1

Body Mind Connection

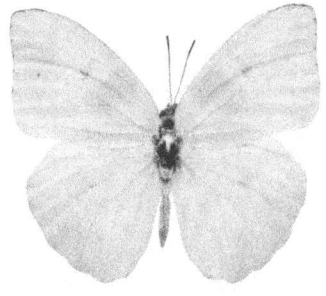

Your thoughts are powerful

World renowned Biology scientist, Dr. Bruce Lipton has discovered that our gene activity can change every day. He says, "If the perception in your mind is reflected in the chemistry of your body, and your nervous system reads and interprets the environment and then controls the blood's chemistry, then you can literally change the fate of your cells by altering your thoughts."

I discovered this truth in my personal epiphany in Hawaii while experts found it scientifically. The truth is the truth, no matter how it is revealed! The integrity of our cells is created from our own perceptions!

Personally, I perceive myself as youthful. I never give "old age" a thought and my cells keep responding to my belief, and because of this, my natural aging process has slowed down! This is the result of the body-mind connection. Dr. Lipton refers to this as: "The Biology of Belief" which is the title of one of his popular books.

The undeniable truth is: Your mind-set is so powerful it can reverse and slow down the aging process, and create health in your entire being, or cause you to age more rapidly and manifest illness. Remember, what you tell yourself everyday will either build you up or tear you down, because your cells are listening!

Belief in your doctor and what he says to you can also create a positive or negative outcome in your body's response. It is a known fact, that sometimes a physician will give a patient a placebo after many tests reveal the person is not really ill, and the patient still won't give up the "self-created idea" of being sick, or having a chronic pain of some kind. After the patient takes the placebo pills with the doctors' firm affirmation they will be cured, the illness or pain symptoms miraculously go away!

The bottom-line is YOU are in charge of what you desire to create! Thoughts are powerful, creative mind symbols! Learn to ignore any doubt that may creep into your ego mind, when your higher intention is to manifest a new way of thinking, and living your life! Doubts usually surface from old beliefs, and past conditioning from life experiences that have taken root in the sub-conscious mind.

Do not offer any energy (thought) to what you don't want! There is an old and true adage that says "what, you focus on expands". Keep your thoughts only on what you want to see happen for your best interest.

To help yourself be ageless and healthy, and to have the life you really want to live, write down your intentions, and as you write, feel it emotionally. Bring the mind and body together in your feeling nature. Next, visualize what you want in your minds' eye, and then speak your intention out-loud. Words carry great energy patterns for establishing the power of belief.

Have faith that your intention is now planted firmly, and that it is in the process of becoming your reality right now. "Now" is all there really is! Begin to live your life positively with full awareness of the present moment, and be open to receive that which you desire. Act as if, it already IS!

Remember, there is no need to "push the river" so resolve to go with the flow and to be open and fully aware that your good is always here, right now. Change your thoughts, change your life. You are the programmer and the director, YOU are it!

Meditation

Meditation is perfect for the body-mind connection. It is the ultimate connection experience. Meditation not only focuses thought and relaxes the brain/mind it lowers blood pressure and balances other vital body functions. Meditation causes a state of wellbeing in the entire system.

Recent clinical (scientific) studies have shown that people who practice meditation tend to live longer with quality of life, due to increased cellular telomerase activity. In fact science is pondering that there may be the possibility that meditation actually slows down biological aging.

A ground breaking study led by Harvard University Neuroscientists, and Massachusetts General Hospital and Boston University, proved by MRI brain scans taken before and after meditation, that positive brain changes took place in their group studies of those who meditated for just eight weeks for 28 minutes each day.

After meditation practice, it was noted that massive changes occurred with an increase in the density of the brains gray matter. Increase in gray matter in the Hippocampus where memory, learning and other cognitive functions occur, was discovered. It also found that meditation synchronized the left and right brain hemispheres. Scientists also learned there was an increased activity of the "prefrontal cortex" of the brain, an area responsible for advanced thinking ability and performance.

Dr. Andrew Newberg Neuroscientist (Oxford University) is one of the leading researchers focused on meditation and the brain. He has explored how meditation helps to relieve stress, improve attention and cognitive abilities, to increase creativity, and to contribute to overall brain health.

Brain scans were also used in people assigned to 8 weeks of "Kirtan Krya" Meditation chant techniques, and it was discovered after 8 weeks of practice, there was positive increased brain function which included memory functions. Scientific studies are now indicating there may be a promise for prevention and/or treatment for Alzheimer's disease, and other forms of brain malfunction, such as dementia by the practice of certain types of meditation techniques, "Kirtan Krya" being one that seems to work well.

KIRTIAN KRYA CHANT
SA TA NA MA

Saying the chant includes bringing the thumb and index fingers together with the first sound of SA and then, all of the fingers following with touching of the thumb each time. Both hands are doing it in unison. The time for the total practice is 8 minutes, and must be done daily for 8 weeks, for results.

2 minutes out-loud

2 minutes whisper

2 minutes thinking it

2 minutes out-loud

I highly suggest that you meditate for creating a strong Body-Mind Connection. When the brain and mind are in coherence there is harmony. Harmony promotes health and agelessness.

Step 2

Your State of Awareness

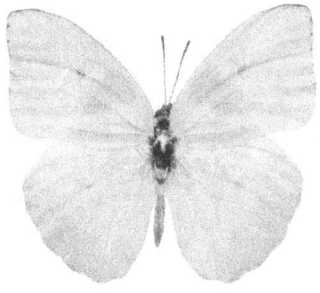

For Positive Life Change,
Open Your Mind Into A State of Awareness with
Consciously Directed Observation

Begin to observe people, starting with seniors.

Make it a point to observe people who are in their fifties
and beyond. You will notice some of them are old before
their time, and that others appear to be vibrant and
young for their chronological age. Chronological age
doesn't matter, in reality age is just a programed illusion
of the mind.

Since age is an illusion in your mind, you can reverse
the aging process regardless of your current age. You can
reset your biological clock back by ten or more years! You
can begin to do it now, by changing your mind-set.

Your old mind-set patterns about aging can be
replaced by the renewing of your mind as we discussed
in the previous section. A fresh mind is youthful because
it is alert, curious, receptive, and filled with thoughts of
new possibilities.

A youthful mind is passionate about life. Living in
full awareness is being passionate about life! Awareness
includes taking in the grandeur and beauty of nature
and appreciating the little things in life that are sweet
and lovely. It is also about gratitude. A youthful mind is

all about heightened awareness, and the excitement of being alive

An open and renewed mind is about love, giving it and receiving it. It is about trusting in the interaction with others, and connecting with them for satisfying and joyful relationships. This can be with your mate, your family and your friends. It is about being vulnerable and going with the flow of life. With an open mind, you will find yourself becoming more adaptable, happier, and spontaneous, moment-by-moment. This is what youth is!

Begin to watch the behavior of children.

See how wonderfully enthusiastic and spontaneous and carefree they are. You can learn a lot from children, as they are so vital and passionate about life. Recall when you were a child, and learn how to re-capture that innocence and that glorious feeling of living in the focused, exciting moment of the NOW.

Do you remember how you used to explore your little world with anticipation and excitement? You wanted to learn about everything, and to touch it, feel it, smell it, and taste it. You were a learner. You were totally trusting and very curious.

The curious mind is a healthy mind, and when you expand your mind through learning and exploring something new, you also exercise it. Exercise is just as important for the mind as it is for the body. This is when you co-partner with your brain. Keep your mind-set young and flexible, and you will be young and flexible. You and your thoughts are one. WHAT YOU THINK, YOU ARE!

Devise a plan to keep learning throughout your life journey. Learn to see life from a new point of view. Be willing to let go of some of your preconceived ideas that you have grown attached to. Let your mind soar into new areas of thought and new dimensions of awareness. Do whatever it takes to get a different perspective of the bigger picture of yourself and your life situation. Learn to view yourself from all different angles. Consider yourself an artist in all aspects of your life and sculpt a new, creative, and exciting life for yourself.

"Satisfaction of one's curiosity is one of the greatest sources of happiness in life"
Linus Pauling

Your feelings are important.

Like a child, be open to your feelings. You may be feeling sunny one day, and hiding behind a gray cloud the next. It is okay to be gloomy once in awhile. After all, there are sunny days and cloudy days, even in nature. Feel everything and develop your emotional sensitivity.

Never bottle up your sad or angry emotions, because if you stuff them, they will surface in negative ways, and often lead to addictions, chronic disease, or other uncomfortable physical conditions. Seek to heal your self emotionally, and learn to handle your feelings wisely and then let them go! Don't allow yourself to vent your negative feelings onto others. Learn to take responsibility for them, for they belong to you! Become fluid like water and open your heart up to all that is life, and to all that you are.

Emotions go beyond feeling up or down. Other feelings you may experience are inner urging's, or sudden hunches. These are called intuition. Paying attention to your "gut instinct" can lead you to an ideal outcome. It is my belief, that intuition is a spiritual experience that needs to be tuned into, and listened to. Children are very open to the subtle prompting's of Spirit, as they have not yet been conditioned to close down their natural perceptions.

Recreate what you loved to do as a child

Children love to play. Finger painting, blowing bubbles and chasing after the magical and ever-elusive rainbow, gives them great joy. They have wonderful imaginations and enjoy playing out their fantasies. Sometimes, they love to lie on the grass and watch the clouds sail by in the blue sky, while imagining them to be dogs, teddy bears, angels, flying saucers, and so forth. They enjoy taking time to just be, and to daydream frequently. So, remember to bring play back into your life. Play is divine re-creation.

"Imagination is more important than knowledge."
Albert Einstein

Laughter is healing and feels so good!

When you laugh, you are in the present moment of sheer delight, and you experience joy, which is true freedom of spirit. Laughter cleanses, releases physical and mental stress, and gives pleasure to the soul. Freeing the spirit through laughter will lead you to your creative passion. In China and in some places in the U.S. there are "yoga laughter" clinics, because laughter heals!

"At the height of laughter, the universe is flung into a kaleidoscope of new possibilities."
Jean Houston

Be a learner.

Resolve to be a learner who loves to explore. Learn to re-develop your zest for discovery, and take a risk now and then by trying something totally new. You might be surprised at how great the new adventure turns out to be.

Children are naturally interested in self-discovery. They are always seeking answers. They want to know the truth about: What is that? How does that work? "Who am I?", "Where did I come from?", and "Why am I here?" There are always many whys! And of course the big question, "Who made God, and who made that, which created God?" Children are very interested in the inner world of how things work, as well as the outer world.

I think, as adults we all still have some of those questions unanswered. Perhaps, you might enjoy seeking the inner world for self-discovery and answers. It is in the stillness that you can find peace, refreshment, renewal and wisdom.

Step 3

Renew The Power
of Your Mind
and Body

Renew The Power of Your Mind and Body by Entering Into Stillness

It is in the quiet inner spaces where you can renew the power of your mind and reverse your biological clock.

It is in the void where all things are possible with Spirit, you can redirect your mind-body intelligence to reset your biological clock, and move time back ten or more years. This space is sacred, and it is where ideas and your innermost desires can be created and nurtured into form.

In the inner spaces of stillness you will feel a sense of peace, as your persistent "mind chatter' releases its' hold on you. The peacefulness of your mind will lead you into a field of unlimited possibilities. Your mind will be clear and bright, and you will feel light, and aware of the mind essence that is present in every cell of your body.

When you experience the mind in and of itself, you will be in touch with the true nature of your being. Your true nature is serene, and free of anxious thoughts. Your true nature knows that all things are possible!

Your body is not just a structure made of flesh. It is a field of mind energy that contains life giving information. Your body knows how to give warning signals when it is out of balance and it knows how to heal itself if you will listen. Your body also knows how to reverse the aging process as well! Your body just needs your awareness and your cooperation. It is in the inner space where you experience full awareness.

In the stillness of your mind, you can transform your body and your life. In the inner spaces of stillness, you can take a quantum leap! In the quantum sphere, an aware observer is required to create a happening or an event. Before a subatomic particle is observed, it exists only as a virtual particle; all events are virtual events until they are consciously observed. This means that you are very powerful. You affect everything you see. Change your perceptions and you will change how and what you see! You will transform yourself!

Lasting self-renewal on any level must be started and maintained at a spiritual level. Without embracing Spirit, a huge piece is missing. Become, as a little child and trust in the creative, loving power of Spirit within you and around you.

Spirit is sometimes referred to as the Unified Field of Consciousness, or Super Consciousness which can be thought of as "creative mind." Spirit, or the Unified Field, whatever you choose to call it is of no consequence. It exists as an infinite field of potential of all possibilities. It knows no limitations. The Unified Field encompasses everything, from the macroscopic to the microscopic. It is all pervasive.

When you become clear about Spirit and the sacred spaces within yourself, (your heart self), hopefully you recognize and acknowledge the limitless power provided to you. With this inner power you can manifest your dreams.

Step 4

Feed Your Cells
With Happiness

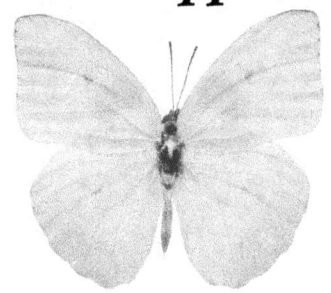

Feed Your Cells With Happiness

Do you really know how to be happy? Happiness doesn't appear by sheer magic however, it is something we can learn to cultivate. But, how can we create the reality of happiness?

Studies by Mayo Clinic reports, about ten percent of people's happiness can be explained by differences in their circumstances. It appears that the bulk of what determines happiness is due to personality, and more importantly thoughts and behaviors that can be changed for the better.

This study tells us that being happy is not always the result from being born with wealth already provided for our life or, from fame or, living an easy lifestyle. People who are truly happy seem to realize that their happiness is the sum of their life choices, and that their lives are built on the positive life decisions such as: Devoting time to family and friends, appreciating what they have right now, maintaining a positive perception about life in general, feeling a sense of purpose, and keeping centered in the present moment.

Basically, happiness seems to stem from our choices, thoughts and actions. Of course we are not always able to be on a happy high because, life seems to hand us challenges out of "the blue" that we need to work through but, we can keep our sense of equanimity during these stressful times. We are capable of being able push our happiness level up a notch due to our conscious perceptions as, to how we view or feel about the situation.

The Trail To A Happier You

Surround yourself with positive people. Nurture all of your relationships, your care for them will be returned with the joy you feel inside for being of service. And, there may be times when those people will be there to support you. This is just the way life works!

Build up your emotional account with kind words and actions. Learn to express gratitude. Gratitude is more than saying, thank you. It is a sense of wonder, appreciation and thankfulness for life itself. It is all too easy to go through life without recognizing your good fortune. Sometimes, it takes a hard knock, such as a serious illness or a loss to jolt people into appreciating the meaningful things in life. Don't wait for that to happen, be in gratitude for what you have in your life now.

Gratitude invites happiness! Make it a daily commitment to practice gratitude. Let it be the first thought and feeling when you open your eyes in the morning and the last thought and feeling, before you retire for the night.

The Scientific American Magazine has carried many articles on how happiness creates a healthy mind/body connection. As far back as 1964 a magazine editor Norman Cousins was diagnosed with a life threatening autoimmune disease, and was given a 1 in 500 chance to recover! Cousins rejected his doctors' prognosis and embarked on his own cure which was happiness thinking! He used laughter and the feeling of happiness, by watching funny movies and so forth, and he completely recovered.

Studies from 1980's and 1990's revealed the brain is directly wired to the immune system, and immune cells have receptors for neurotransmitters, suggesting that there is cross communication. Studies revealed since that time, have consistently shown the power of the mind in a" happy state", breeds happy cells! So, don't worry, be happy! The end result can be good health and agelessness!

Quotes About Happiness

"Be happy for this moment. This moment is your life."
   Omar Khyyam

"Happiness is not something ready made. It comes from your own actions".
   Dali Lama

"Happiness is when, what you think and what you say, and what you do are all in harmony."
   Mathatma Gandhi

Find Your Purpose

People who strive to meet a goal, whether it is creating a painting, writing a book, running in a marathon, growing a garden, caring for children, teaching or learning something, starting a new business, finding their true belief system, are much happier than those that don't find something they love to do, and are passionate about.

Having a specific goal for each day and for long term provides a sense of purpose and bolsters self esteem. What your personal goal is doesn't matter as much as the process of working toward it, and then accomplishing it. Purpose adds meaning, passion, and joy to life.

Are You Engaged In Doing Something You Love To Do Now?

If not, ask yourself these questions to help you discover your purpose:
- **What excites me and energizes me?**
- **What are my proudest achievements?**
- **How do I want others to remember me?**

Living Moment To Moment

Don't postpone what you are passionate about, find your joy and live it. Don't make excuses that you are too busy or stressed, and that you can't begin now.

Life will always be busy, so that day may never come for you. Instead look for and enjoy the small pleasures in life every day. Learn to focus on the moment....be here now! When you are here now and in awareness of the present time, your purpose will come into focus. Happiness is finding your joy...your purpose! It is being in relationship with all of life!

The fleeting moments of joy, spending time at parties,

going to movies, going on a trip and so forth, welcoming new life into the world, and celebrating all different kinds of occasions add to your state of happiness. These parts help to make up the whole.

Each person comes into life to fulfill a special destiny. There is a purpose for your life. Find what you love to do, and simply do it!

Quotes About Purpose

"When you are inspired by some great purpose, some extraordinary project, all your thoughts break their bonds: your mind transcends limitations, your consciousness expands in every direction and you find yourself in a new, great and wonderful world. Dormant forces, faculties and talents become alive, and you discover yourself to be a greater person by far than you ever dreamed yourself to be".
Pantanjali

"The purpose of life is to live it, to taste the experience to the ultimate, to reach out eagerly and without fear for a newer and richer experience."
Eleanor Roosevelt

"It is in your moments of decision that your destiny is shaped."
Tony Robbins

Step 5

How to De-Stress Yourself

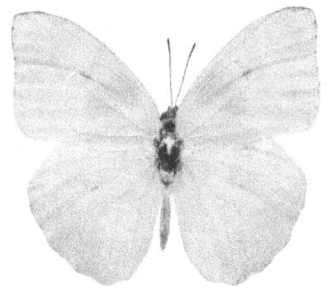

How To "De-Stress Yourself"

Learning How to manage your stress levels promotes agelessness.

As a certified stress management consultant, as well as teaching how to be ageless, I have found that many of my clients and groups that I have addressed through speaking and presenting workshops, do not know how to deal effectively with their stress. Too much stress causes aging and illness, and this is a known medical fact.

First of all, it is your individual responsibility to take charge of managing your stress. Self value and realizing you are in control of your life responses to all situations is a good beginning point. This means that you are in charge of your perceptions, thoughts, and emotions on how you deal with challenges. It is the basic understanding that experience is not what happens to you, it is what you do with, what happens to you.

Complete elimination of stress in your life is unrealistic. In fact, we all need some tension to motivate us! But, it is important to identify major stressors in your work, and your personal life. First of all, learn to accept what is, and then personally plan how to reduce those stress factors. Learning to make and apply "on the spot" or, "real time," stress reducers is the key to stress management.

Real time stress management is as easy as pausing and tuning into your breath and breathing deeply from your belly, while slowly drawing the air into your lungs, and then gently releasing it through slightly parted lips. This highly effective and easy breath exercise should be repeated at least three times in a row, and ten times is better. It depends on your situation. You can do this anywhere and at anytime.

Another easy stress reducer is to isolate and tense the muscles of your shoulders, squeeze tightly ten times and then let go, to relax them. Check your shoulders during the day to see if you have them pulled up, or if they are down in a normal position.

Make room in your day often, to move and stretch your body, especially if you sit a lot. Conscious and frequent movement of some type for your body, reduces stress, relaxes the mind, and creates more energy.

Mindful Meditation has become a popular technique for relaxation. Mindful Meditation focuses on the breath in the present moment. This method of reducing stress also encompasses focus on the outer space surroundings, as well as the inner space.

When we are in full awareness of the moment we resonate with the Body-Mind connection, and this is when we can relax and be with "what is." We are not thinking about the past or the future when focused on the Now. The past represents the last moment and the future is the next moment.

You can reduce stress on a nature walk, or a walk around your block. You can notice spaces and yet the wholeness of your environment. For example, the next time you are on a walk and see a tree, notice the whole tree, and then focus on its parts. As you observe the tree notice the spaces and designs within and around the tree, and then focus your attention on the detailed patterns of the bark. Continue being in the focused moment with the tree, taking in the branches, and all the little intricacies. This is a great way to reduce stress, as your mind is completely on the tree, and not thinking about the past, or future moments! You can choose to do this mindful meditation anytime and anywhere with anything, even staring at a candle flame or, a dancing fire in the fireplace.

UCLA and many other prestigious colleges across the country are offering Mindful Meditation techniques to their students, especially to those that are studying medicine. The medical profession is now being made aware of how Mindful Meditation can reduce pain and relieve depression, without traditional medication.

For long term stress management, check over your total lifestyle, and resolve to make positive changes. You will then, be able to live a more relaxing, happy and healthy life for yourself. If you have problems following a plan, then see a stress management consultant, or therapist.

Choosing Resilience

In the school of life we need to learn to be resilient in order to manage our stress levels. When we are flexible the ability to handle difficult situations is increased, and we are able to act from the core of our being where our inner strength resides. Resilience also means that we are open to reaching out to others for the help and support we require. When we are authentic with our feelings and needs we are being true and compassionate to ourselves, and this is a sign of inner power.

Resilience also means that we are fully aware of the present moment, for in the "Now" clear decisions can be made.

According to psychological and social studies resilience means, positive adaptation to negative conditions that can be associated with natural disasters, losses of all kinds, tragedy, and even forced confinement over long periods of time.

For an example of resilience: Nelson Mandela South African antiapartheid revolutionary who served as President, and endured twenty-seven years of prison with hard labor for trying to free South Africa, was able to maintain his equanimity. He consistently kept his optimistic attitude and his vision alive for being released in the future, even though there was no evidence of it.

While still imprisoned he wrote a letter to his children before he was finally released. "One day I will look back. I will be home to live in happiness until the end of my days." When he was released the whole world watched and was amazed at his resilience.

Resources for help

Counseling by a certified counselor or spiritual/religious advisor may help you to let go of emotional baggage if trying self-help techniques does not work for you. Reaching out for help means you care about yourself!

Alternative Therapies such as Acupressure, Acupuncture, Massage, Chiropractic, and other hands on techniques, such as, Touch for Health, and Reiki, are often able to help in the release of "old stuff" that manifests in the body, such as pain, stiffness and disease.

Yoga

A popular Ancient Exercise, now practiced and fully accepted in the modern world is Hatha Yoga for health and well-being, and it is excellent for helping to release blocks of energy that are caught in the body.

As a certified Hatha Yoga Instructor, I can attest that yoga can help to release old baggage and bring emotional and physical resilience into your awareness. Yoga emphasizes physical postures, deep slow breathing and holding or, fluid movements. It is noted for improving brain functions such as cognition and focus, as well as boosting the memory at any age. When you practice yoga it is definitely a body-mind connection. Yoga should be practiced at least several times a week for the greatest benefit.

According, to the National Center for Complementary Alternative Medicine, in Bethesda, Maryland, they have been using MRI Scans on groups of people that have been practicing yoga regularly, and it was found they exhibited more gray matter brain cells, as compared to those people who did not practice the art of yoga. When practicing Yoga the body must conform to the thinking process on how to accomplish different and precise movements.

Yoga is also known to dramatically reduce stress levels. It can lower blood pressure, reduce harmful cholesterol levels, increase bone density, increase lung capacity, help lower blood sugars in diabetics, and improve heart function. It helps maintain normal weight, releases pain in the neck, back and shoulders. Yoga strengthens the legs and arms and entire body, and flexibility is definitely increased along with balance!

According to Dr. Paula Chu she wrote, in the December 2014 issue of the European Journal of Preventative Cardiology, "We believe there is promising evidence on the effect of Yoga on improving cardiovascular risk factors." Yoga practice definitely promotes health and Agelessness!

A preliminary study involving 75 sedentary adults with rheumatoid arthritis or knee osteoarthritis found that an 8 week yoga program (two classes per week and one more home practice) resulted in physical health, psychological health and overall physical activity. Because much of these benefits were still evident nine months later and no yoga related adverse events were recorded, the authors of the study note that yoga may help sedentary adults with arthritis to safely increase their physical activity levels. Journal of Rheumatology, April 2015.

Tai Chi

Tai Chi is also growing in popularity in the Western world. It involves certain fluid movements for balance. Tia Chi strengthens the legs and promotes the flow of vital energy through the body. It calms the mind, and helps to restore balance to the entire body systems through the mind-body connection. In the practice of Tai Chi (as in Yoga) you have to "think" as your body moves in new ways! This is the body-mind connection. Tia Chi is great for any age, but especially for seniors who want to improve their balance.

General Exercise

Move your body into motion daily! If Yoga or Tai Chi does not appeal to you, choose an exercise that you know you will do on a regular basis.

If you are a senior low impact exercise is a good choice, along with a regular walking routine to get your heart rate up.

General western exercise methods offered by Fitness Clubs are also good choices. Exercising by swimming, dancing, bicycling, playing tennis, anything that moves you into action, and involves the body-mind connection, is a must for being ageless! Any regular exercise not only increases muscle tone and body strength, the routine also increases brain power, which helps ward off brain degeneration.

Step 6

A Healthy Diet

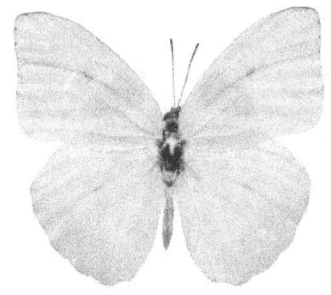

A Healthy Diet Means
A Healthier and Younger You

We have all heard about how we need to eat right in order to be energetically healthy and to keep our weight balanced in regards to our frame and height.

As we approach mid-life, we do not metabolize our food as quickly as we did in our younger years. This, of course, means that we are not well equipped to burn up those calories. A slow metabolism means we store more body fat!

If we eat right and take the correct supplements, we can actually reset our metabolic rate. While exercise is a huge factor, lessening caloric intake is also important. Never go on a crash diet, no matter what your age is! Learn to eat sensibly, and eat smaller portions.

Consider this rule of thumb: only 30 percent of your calories should come from fat.

Eat red meat only once a week if you enjoy it, and shop for organically fed beef, or lean free-range beef. White meat such as chicken or turkey, fish, and a few organic eggs a week should give you all the protein you need. Always buy free-range poultry and wild caught fish. Sardines that are canned are another fish you may consider using frequently, as sardines are thought to be food for the brain! I buy the skinless and boneless variety that is packed in water and low in sodium. I make sure the fish is cold, and then I squeeze lemon over them. They are a mild fish.

Eat several servings a week of foods prepared from lentils, dried peas, beans, brown or wild rice, and barley, Always use whole grains for your breads, cereals and pastas, unless you need to use gluten free products. These are whole foods and contain significant amounts of fiber.

Go heavy on fresh or frozen vegetables and fruits. Canned goods lose much of their vitality. Remember, 'an apple a day, keeps the doctor away!' Always consume as many different colors for your vegetables and fruits as possible. In addition, don't forget the berries and dark plums! Blueberries and dark plums are considered to be brain food!

Buy organic food when you can. Most of my food is organic. I feel naturally grown food is keeping me free of toxins from pesticides, irradiation, genetically altered components, and depleted soils. Depleted soils rob the plants and trees of natural, enriched elements. Organic food is naturally healthful and preventative. I do everything I possibly can to be well now, and in the years to come.

Dairy products are also important. Use cheese (including cottage cheese) in moderation. If milk agrees with you, consume it too, but buy organic milk as other milk is usually treated with Bovine Growth hormones.. If you cannot tolerate animal milks, try almond, rice, or organic soymilk. It is also a good idea to take extra calcium with magnesium and zinc for healthy teeth and bones.

Step 7

Vital Supplements

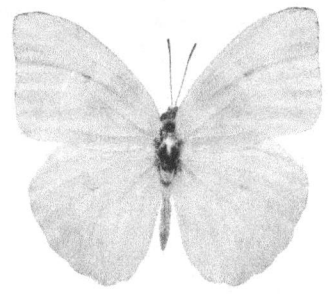

Supplements are Vital for
Maintaining Health and Youth

Vitamins, minerals, and herbal supplements are important in your dietary plan.

Notice: If you have a health condition, consult with your doctor before following my suggestions for supplements and herbs.

If you could look inside my kitchen cupboard, you would find bottle after bottle of vitamins, minerals, and herbal supplements. You would perhaps exclaim, "I could never swallow all of those pills!" Well, if I can, you can. Believe me, they make a huge difference in my overall energy level, and help to keep my body from rapid aging.

I have developed an anti-aging supplement regimen, and it is working alongside everything else I am doing.

I am not on any medication at age eighty-two. My blood pressure is 110 over 60 most of the time, and my body is quite relaxed and happy, as I do not carry around pain. This equates to agelessness. I am happy and my body follows my feeling!

When my cholesterol was a bit high about ten years ago, my doctor wanted to put me on a Statin drug. I refused. I told him I would come back for another test in six months and that my cholesterol would be in a normal range. He agreed, knowing how I preferred to deal naturally with my health issues.

I ate oat bread and natural oat cereals. I began to take a non-flush niacin pill daily, which I knew to be crucial in helping to lower the cholesterol rate. I reduced my fat intake as well. I walked for longer periods of time. Within the six-month period per our agreement, I had another test done. It was in the normal range. I gave my doctor an education as to how cholesterol can be lowered naturally. He was quite impressed!

Here are some suggested supplements for wellness and anti-aging:

Resveratrol

Have you heard of the newest anti-aging supplement? It is called Resveratrol. Currently I am taking 3 ounces of it daily. It tastes great! In liquid form, it is potent and is easily absorbed. Each one-ounce serving is equal to the benefits of 1,300 glasses of red wine! Multiply that by three servings and I am taking in the benefits of 3,900 glasses of wine a day...all with no hangover! The guidelines suggest one to three ounces daily. This compound is a natural antioxidant. Resveratrol also comes in capsules. For years, researchers have studied resveratrol, linking it to reduced risk of cancer, heart disease, and brain diseases such as Alzheimer's, and some other diseases that are more prevalent in people as time goes by.

Researchers have been very busy trying to identify substances that influence age-regulating genes. It appears resveratrol may be one of them. Harvard studies show that resveratrol may be able to assist cells in living longer and healthier life spans. Since we are composed of cells, this includes us!

Turmeric (root extract)

Turmeric is an antioxidant that works inside the cells. Turmeric has anti-cancer components and it has powerful anti-inflammatory properties for joints. It reduces inflammation in the entire body. I have taken Turmeric capsules and cooked with this spice faithfully for over 8 years, and I do not experience aches and pains that plague most people. It is thought to be good for arthritis.

Cayenne Pepper

Cayenne is thought to be a powerful herb (which is often used in spicy cooking). It also comes in capsules, extracts, and teas. It is thought to have been successfully used for warding off heart attacks, helping heart attack recovery, or even stopping a heart attack in that moment! I cannot personally attest to this, I have only read about the healing properties of Cayenne on the Internet, and I cannot endorse it. Cayenne pepper is also used to settle stomach discomfort and to aid in the digestive process, and more. You may wish to do an Internet search on the benefits of Cayenne. You may come across testimonies about heart conditions…as I did when I researched this spice and herb.

Green tea

Green tea has powerful antioxidant properties. Green tea is thought to be anti-aging and fights free radicals, which cause cells to mutate causing cancer and other diseases. Green tea may be beneficial for the heart and may help to ward off a stroke. Three to six cups of green tea per day are recommended, but taking 3 capsules a day is a lot eaiser to consume on a regular basis than drinking tea all day! I take the capsules.

Ginkgo Biloba

Many people have reported that after taking this herbal supplement, their mental clarity, and memory improved. This herb may thin your blood, so ask your doctor about it, before consuming this herb. Ginkgo Biloba should be deleted 10 days before any surgery, as it can cause more bleeding to occur, as can Vitamin E, fish oils, and aspirin.

Flax oil or Salmon Fish oil soft-gels (or liquid forms)

It is thought that taking this oil provides you with potent Omega 3's for increased brain power, it also assists in reducing inflammation, and helps to prevent cardiovascular disease.

Acidophilus (milk free) capsules or liquid

Acidophilus adds friendly bacteria to the colon and helps to establish a healthy digestive system.

Digestive Enzymes

These aid your body in digestion and maximize the absorption of nutritional elements. There are many options; ask your doctor or health food store advisor to assist you.

Phytonutrients

Phytonutrients are the biological substances that give vegetables and fruits their colors, smells and flavors.

These properties are natural antioxidants, and help to prevent diseases and body imbalances. They help with slowing the aging process. It is recommended that we consume plant foods from each color of the rainbow daily. Since this is difficult for a lot of people, there is a powdered version that you can add to juices. I take a product called "Vibrant Health." This powder contains a full spectrum of color and is equivalent to 4 to 5 servings of fresh fruits and vegetables. There are other brands available.

Spirulina

This dark green sea powder promotes healthy eyes, supports the immune system, assists in maintaining balanced cholesterol levels, increases cellular health and creates more energetic feelings.

Dark Chocolate

Dark chocolate candy is thought to help lower bad cholesterol and to be rich in antioxidants. Seven ounces a week is recommended, which is one ounce per day. You can use the organic version or non-organic, your choice. I use either one. Be sure your chocolate is at least 70 percent cacao and dark!

About garlic

Garlic acts as a superior tonic for the cardiovascular system. In addition it acts as a strong antiseptic counteracting the growth of harmful bacteria in the body. It also boosts the immune system and is thought to ward off cancer, since it inactivates some of the carcinogens that we ingest daily. It also thought to protect the DNA from degenerative changes. Garlic is available in capsule form.

B3 (niacin)

Niacin is available in a non-flush version. This is helpful in reducing harmful cholesterol, and is great for the skin and more!

More about Vitamins and Minerals

It is wise to take a 'one-a-day' combination of vitamins and minerals. Be certain you include extra calcium with magnesium. Vitamin C and Vitamin D are especially important, as well as a B complex. I take a multi-vitamin with minerals, and then add more of the C, D, and B vitamins. You can overdose on vitamin B. Talk to your physician, or health food advisor or nutritionist, before adding more supplements to your multi-vitamin and minerals.

Chia Seeds

Is This A Miracle Food?

Chia was first used as a food as early as 3500 by the Aztecs, and later by the South West Indians. Chia has an ancient and valid history.

Chia is said to be the richest plant source of the essential Omega-3 fatty acids and it contains natural antioxidants. It is also verified as a high-energy endurance food. It was used by the Aztec warriors while they were on long marches to do battle, and. they subsisted on Chia seeds during their conquests.

Historians have documented, the South West Indians would eat as little as a tablespoon of Chia seeds per day when they were on long, forced marches to keep their energy levels up. Chia expands in the intestines, especially when water is taken, and so they didn't feel like they were starving. Indians running from the Colorado River to the California coast to trade turquoise for seashells, would only bring Chia seeds for their main source of nourishment.

Chia seeds are regenerators for the cells and the muscles and tissues. Perhaps these seeds are the definitive hydrophilic colloid for the 21st century diet! The hydrophilic colloids are known to form the underlying elements of all living cells.

Hydrophilic colloids possess the property of readily taking up and giving off the substances essential to cell life.

Chia is also rich in calcium as it contains the mineral boron, which acts as a catalyst for absorption of the calcium by the body. Chia has a vast array of other vitamins and minerals. Chia is digested and absorbed easily by the body.

For slimming and trimming, Chia seeds are helpful for reducing those unwanted pounds!

These seeds can assist you in loosing weight for two reasons. The first reason being, they are so filling that you will consume less food. The second reason is that your body will be cleansed of toxic junk that has built up in your intestines. Chia is a fiber and your colon health will be assisted by this natural bulk. Be sure to drink extra water after taking these seeds!

Never use Chia Pet seeds! These seeds are contaminated with pesticides. Purchase your seeds from your Health Food Store, or by ordering from a website that sells organic products.

Do your own research on this health food, there is a lot of information available in books and of course on websites, then you will make a good choice for yourself.

A word of CAUTION: if you have a health problem that requires you to take medication, be certain to check with your health care professional before you take herbal supplements. Herbs are natural medicines, and can interact in a harmful way with some medications!

Step 8

Water Intake

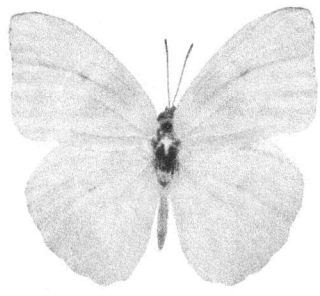

The importance of water

Some people may forget to drink enough water.

As we progress in years, our body's message to drink water sometimes lessens in strength. This is when dehydration, illness and finally a premature death can set in.

We discussed earlier what certain foods and supplements can do for keeping your brain- mind youthful and clear. Another way to have a good memory is to keep your brain hydrated by drinking six to eight glasses of water a day. Your brain tissue needs water, just like your body tissue does!

Think of a desert. Long periods of drought create cracks in the soil where nothing can grow and flourish. You would die of dehydration in a desert without water. Now think of a tropical forest, where there is an abundance of water. In the tropical forest, every thing is plump, lush and flourishing with life. Your brain needs water as does your body, so that you can flourish. Your body is your personal environment.

When you were born, you were 80 percent water!

The water level of your cells dropped as you matured, and at a healthy adult stage, you are about 70 percent water. Make certain you maintain that healthy level of hydration! Water also detoxifies your system so, a healthy intake of water is crucial for many reasons.

How much water should you consume each day?

There is a formula you can use to guide you as to how many cups a day your body needs.

Take your current weight and divide it by 2, that will give you your total. For instance if you weigh 160 pounds that will be 80 ounces or 10 cups of water a day! Eight ounces times 10 equals 80. Other beverages don't count. Drinking enough water helps to reverse aging!

It is a wise person that takes a bottle of water with them where ever they go, as sometimes our outings put us in places where we cannot access water when we need it. Getting in the habit of taking water with you will also remind you to drink!

Never leave your water in a plastic bottle in your car, or where it can get warm or hot as it can leech harmful chemicals from the plastic into your water.

Water purification systems

It is wise to have some kind of good water purifying system for your everyday drinking water. Some water units may be cost prohibitive. Even something like a Brita™ pitcher with water-purifying filter refills, is better than drinking most water straight out of the tap. Do your own research so that you can make a wise decision about getting a water filtering system that will fit your budget and lifestyle. (Buyer beware!) Do extensive research before investing in a costly water purification system!

Step 9

Sleep and Rest

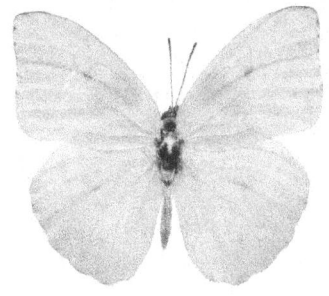

The Importance of Deep Sleep and Restful Periods

Deep sleep promotes health and youthfulness.

When you get a good night's rest, your body renews itself in many different ways. Sleep is essential for healthy cell growth, and for cell and tissue repair. Sleep boosts the immune system. During the time we are sleeping, the body's cells increase production, while proteins break down at a slower rate.

Deep sleep enables the brain to encode and store recently received information. REM sleep activates the parts of the brain that deal with learning. Also, during sleep various parts of the brain slow down, including the parts of the brain that control emotions, decision-making, and social interaction. Without sufficient sleep, people are less effective at learning new skills or retaining/recalling information.

Neurons in the brain are related to the nervous system. They also rejuvenate and repair during sleep, so the body can function effectively, physically, mentally, and emotionally.

I suggest that at least an hour before your bedtime that you begin to settle your pace of activity. It is not a good idea to watch something on TV that over stimulates the emotions, or to exercise. The best thing to do for a good nights rest is to prepare for bed leisurely and to read, meditate, and to listen to restful music or recorded sounds of the ocean or rain before retiring. If you have trouble falling asleep after trying all of the above suggestions, follow your breath and think or visualize soft blue. A dark room is the best for sleep.

More information about the importance of restful sounds.

Restful sounds usually help to induce deep sleep in most people. Music can have a tremendously relaxing effect on our minds and bodies. Soft, flowing classical music is particularly good. This type of music can have a profound effect on your physiological functions. It can slow down the heart rate, lower your blood pressure and decrease your levels of stress hormones. It subdues anxious thoughts and soothes the nervous system. Equally beneficial are nature sounds, such as ocean waves, bubbling streams and rainfall. These sounds can take you into a state of timelessness that promotes sleep.

Meditation is restful awareness.

Meditating on a regular basis creates harmony and restfulness in the body and mind. Studies have shown that those who meditate daily, even for ten minutes, are younger biologically than their chronological age. Meditation takes the meditator into a state of timelessness. Meditation is "restful awareness." Studies have shown that DHEA levels are higher in those who meditate. DHEA hormone levels diminish as people age.

It is certainly apparent that restful awareness promotes youth and wellness! Regular periods for meditation will create harmony that lasts, so that by bedtime sleep happens easily and naturally.

Step 10

Hormones and Cellular Functions

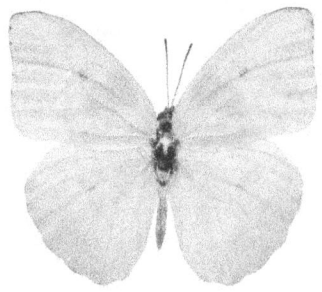

Understanding Your Hormones and Cellular Functions

DHEA is the most common hormone and is known as the master of all hormones.

It is the precursor to over fifty hormones in the body. DHEA is produced in the adrenal glands, and is converted on command to specific hormones the body needs to maintain bodily functions. DHEA is also responsible for producing hormones that control fat and mineral metabolism, as well as managing stress. Overall, it is responsible for maintaining youthful vigor.

DHEA levels can be tested through a Naturopathic Clinic. Usually hair or saliva samples are tested for the DHEA levels. I had my saliva tested, and I take what is called 7-KETO, which boosts my metabolism. I suggest you never use DHEA supplements without a test first. Keep in mind as we take on the higher numbers in years, our DHEA levels become lower! Getting your levels checked may prove to be helpful to your entire body.

DNA and the Genetic Code as it relates to your cells

DNA contains the instructions needed for an organism (YOU) to develop, survive, and reproduce. DNA (double helix strands) is found in a special area of the cells called the nucleus.

During cell division, DNA unwinds so it can be copied, and the copies are transformed to new cells. At the end of the strands of DNA there are cap endings or chains called telomeres.

At birth, human telomeres are long, and as the years pass, eventually the telomeres become so shortened that the losses in replication (copies) begin to affect the DNA sequence, ultimately preventing the cell from being able to duplicate itself correctly. This loss causes body imbalances, aging, and finally death, as more and more cells are unable to copy themselves due to shortened and thin telomeres.

DNA repression

Repression happens when certain genes (genomes) are "shut off," and unable to send out the chemical messages to perform various duties to the cell. Repression can be caused by various factors such as nutritional deficiencies, toxic overload from alcohol consumption, cigarette smoking, and assimilation of food pesticides and/or toxic chemical exposure.

Taking good care not abuse your body and avoiding overindulgences of all kinds, will keep your cells functioning at healthy levels. Using preventative measures will pay off in the long run.

Sometimes, the genetic code that is inherited can cause repression of cells. I believe, by using positive mental habits and taking care of the emotions and body, you can help to break a genetic code that is in your family gene pool. Because, cancer or another disease has been experienced by a family member, does not mean that you will experience it. The safe thing to do is to keep up on your yearly physicals, which includes lab tests and periodic screening for colon and breast cancer, and other health conditions that may exist in your gene bank. This is common sense. Learn to focus on health, not what is in your genetic pool. Do what you can do to make yourself feel good. Be happy and spread your joy!

Step 11

Light From Your Cells

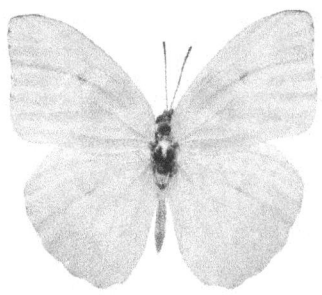

Photons (Light) Are Emitted From Your Cells

Science tells us that photons are quantum electromagnetic energy.

We emit photons (light) from our DNA. In the early 1980's a team of scientists demonstrated that the cells of all living beings emit photons at a rate of approximately 100 units per second and per square centimeter of surface area. They also showed that DNA was the source of this photon emission. Our DNA is sending out messenger particles from our body, in the form of angles of light.

Wikipedia states:

"In physics, the photon is an elementary particle, the quantum of the electromagnetic field and the basic unit of light and all forms of electromagnetic radiation."

Earth science studies by NASA on Green, shows how photons stimulate the growth of plant life and explains that the photon system (which is cosmic light from above), touches the chemical of earth, acting as a powerful energy booster. Since we are "earth beings," it stands to reason that our cells emit light, because photons enter our bodies from the cosmic light rays, as well.

Cosmic rays then, are the light streams of high-energy charged particles, from outer space.

In the Bible, God said; "Let there be light and there was light"

I believe there is the outer light and inner Light. The inner Light is the spiritual Light, the very essence of Higher Being. Jesus used the Light of God (Spirit) to heal others. Light is continually mentioned in the Bible.

Since light has always been with us, light has fascinated philosophers and scientists for centuries! For example, Aristotle studied the components and action of light, and believed that light traveled in waves. Euclid claimed that light traveled in straight lines.

Isaac Newton was documented as the first scientist to discover that by using a prism, light is actually a spectrum of rainbow colors. We give credit to Ole Roemer, who in 1676 was the first to measure the velocity of light.

Even before these discoveries, great philosophers, and physicians such as Hippocrates. the father of medicine, claimed that the eyes, as they absorbed light, were the bridge to the pathway of the entire being, which includes the soul.

I meditate on the physical light (photons) of my DNA and the spiritual Light. Personally, it is my belief we are a combination of physical (body) and spiritual (soul) components. In step 13 of this book, I will reveal some of the steps that I use to bring youth and vitality into my body, by working with the spiritual Light in my cellular structure. Some of the information you may agree with and some you may not. I ask only that you keep an open mind as I share the information with you. This method works for me, and I received a lot of this information from Spirit while in Hawaii.

Step 12

Your DNA

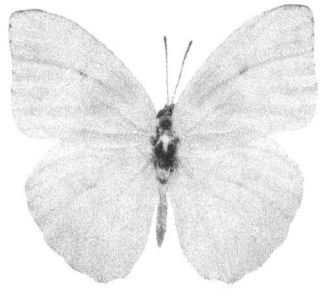

DNA *as it Relates to*
the Pineal Gland for Agelessness,

In the Bible there is a verse that says, "The light of the body is in the eye: if therefore thine eye be single, thy whole body shall be filled with light." The verse does not state 'eyes,' but rather the singular 'eye.' Matthew 6: 22.

You have heard many people express that the "eyes are the windows of the soul." I have used this expression and perhaps you have too.

There is another eye, called the pineal gland. It is pine coned shaped and is known as the single eye or, 'third eye' deep within the center section of the brain. The exact location is between the two hemispheres and behind and above the pituitary gland. If you take your index fingers of both hands and put them directly behind the top of your ears, as they are pointed inward toward the brain, the pineal gland is in the center of that line. In India, red circle marks are used to acknowledge the single eye just above the root of the nose.

The pineal gland receives light from the eyes. Daylight, given to us from the sun, is absorbed into our eyes and it stimulates the activity of the pineal gland.

The pineal gland has many vital functions for keeping the body balanced by using light-related messages that it releases into the body. It also receives information and light bounced back from our internal biological clock. The clock is situated within the hypothalamus. The hypothalamus is located below the thalamus, and above the brain stem. Working in concert with the hypothalamus, the pineal gland knows when to release the hormone melatonin that balances the natural rhythms of the body. I don't want to get into all of the other duties of this gland that is so vital to our body, because I have another point to make.

The hypothalamus and the pineal gland work together in partnership with the receiving and distribution of light in the body. The hypothalamus can be compared to a central receiving station for incoming information also; it acts as the director for sending the information where it needs to go. It maintains the body's harmony, like the conductor of a symphony who keeps all of the musicians synchronized.

The pituitary is another gland, known as the master gland of the body. All of these key glands are in the brain and work together in operating the body. They are the keys to the endocrine system, but are also only a part of other major glands that play the important roles that keep the body in harmony.

The hypothalamus, as the cup of the biological clock, acts as the conductor for the body-mind connection. It contains a key to our aging or agelessness! Remember, it is in concert with the pineal gland and they both receive and direct light, which activates the biological clock.

The telomeres of the DNA are also coded with a light key for resetting the biological clock within the DNA for life extension and agelessness.

In summary, light enters the eyes to serve our vision, but it does much more, as it also stimulates the pineal gland, and then proceeds directly to the body's biological clock in the hypothalamus. The hypothalamus, in turn, sends light-coded information to the pineal gland, or "the third eye" which is another commonly used name for this magnificent single eye gland. The internal clock registers, day-to-night and night-to-day as the years click by. Science has recently found the DNA telomeres also hold a key for life extension and compliment the work of the higher glands.

If we treat our body with respect and nourish it properly, we will enhance our cellular health and longevity. If we abuse our body we can expect ill health, and we will create an untimely old body, and perhaps an early death. We were intended to live very long, healthy and youthful lives.

So, the abuse we do to our bodies is what interrupts the natural health and longevity of our DNA. Toxins build up and the DNA has a more difficult time copying its perfect cellular structure. This is when aging accelerates. Our negative thoughts and a stress filled life also cause faster aging in our cellular structure.

Genetics can play a part in the inherited propensity to certain diseases and how fast we age, but we can alter genetics by a healthy lifestyle that includes positive thinking and a strong connection to Spirit.

I feel that our bodies are completely maintained by Spirit. We are not just an automated machine, made of flesh, blood, bone, tissue and complex systems, operating of its' own accord. If our eye is single, our body is filled with light. This means Spirit's Light, the Light of the world. We have the power to activate that spiritual Light, reverse the aging process, and become ageless. It just takes awareness and reverence for that great life-giving force we call Spirit. We were meant to live at least one hundred years or more, and in good health.

Step 13

Effective Meditation

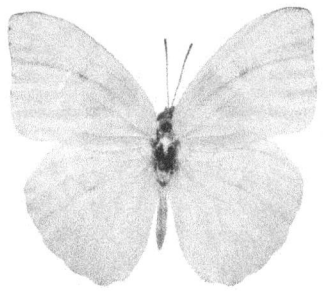

Effective Meditation for Reversing the Aging Process and Resetting Your Biological Clock

I used the following meditation while walking by the sea in Hawaii.

I breathed in not only the sea air, but light coded information as well. I seemed to automatically know that for youthful regeneration, I needed to tune into Spirit by centering my attention into my Pineal Gland, (the Spirit filled) all-seeing eye of wisdom and Light. It was from this sacred space that my age reversal began.

To strengthen your connection with Spirit for a more youthful and healthy YOU, make yourself comfortable in a quiet place. For a sitting and prayerful meditation, sit up straight and put your palms upward on your lap, or you can do a walking prayer and meditation in nature.

Say a prayer to Spirit in your own way, so that you build a loving heart connection. A loving and nurturing mind-set is vital. Spirit is the very essence of love, and Spirit creates in love.

If you are of the Christian, Jewish, or of any Eastern, or New Thought faith, you may alter the words used, or even the method if you need to. Visualization and communicating with your cells is most important! Stay in the comfort zone of your belief system.

Talk to Spirit about your intention, and ask for your desire of agelessness to be given unto you as you co-partner together. "Ask and you will receive."

~ ~ ~

After your prayer, take in a few deep breaths, and as you take these breaths, begin visualizing a brilliant, crystal clear white light that is centered in your pineal gland (the single eye), the chalice for spiritual light coded information. Breathe in light from that point and focus your intention for agelessness, and the biological age you wish to be...into your single eye.

When you are ready, in your minds eye, release the light coded information into your entire head and brain, and let it travel down your neck and along the entire spinal column.

Visualize your spine filled with brilliant white Light, and feel the warmth of loving energy pulsating along your spinal column. Visualize billions of energetic lights literally lighting up the cells of DNA along your spine.

Breathe again into the single eye and focus your attention there once more. Allow the Light to transfer itself, into your face, throat, chest, abdomen, and the pelvis, bring it down your front legs, to your feet. Feel the Light being activated as billions of tiny lights inside every cell, and tissue, fluid, organ and glands of your body, and especially in your heart.

Bring your attention once more into the single eye, and when you are ready breathe the Light down the back of your neck, covering your shoulders, your upper back, arms, hands, your lower back and your buttocks, and all the way down the back of your legs to the heels of your feet. Again, feel the warmth of the spiritual energy and visualize billions of tiny lights popping on...which is the activation of your DNA in sync for regeneration.

Affirm that your DNA is now dividing and copying itself perfectly, and that any cell that has not been dividing normally is now corrected. Affirm that every cell is always in alignment, perfect and whole and filled with the Light of Spirit.

Finally, speak words of agelessness directly to the telomeres at the end of the DNA chromosomes, (visualize them as points of Light) and tell them to restore any damage to themselves, so that they are long and healthy once again and filled with the Light of Spirit.

Continue to be in the silence and just be aware of the Light that has been activated all through your body. Feel the energy of spiritual love pulsating in every cell of your physical self, and continue to breathe in the white Light of Spirit.

When you are ready, reaffirm the new biological age of your choice and consciously tap into the feeling of youth and vitality.

~ ~ ~

I suggest you do this Light coded meditation daily, or at least several times a week and incorporate it as a part of your regular meditation practice. This meditation is a vital piece for reversing the aging process. It IS the Fountain of Youth!

Step 14

Transformational Mirror Talk

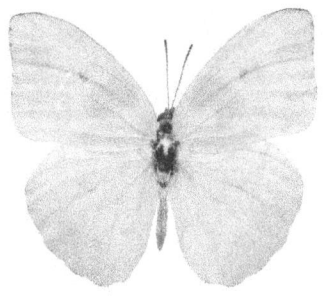

Transformational Mirror Talk

Did you know that talking to yourself while looking into your mirror image can give you an entire new and positive perception about being ageless? Well trust me it can, and does!

After receiving the spiritual downloaded information about being ageless while I was in Hawaii in 2008, I was also intuitively guided to do mirror image "self-talk." Mirror talk is related to silent meditation, (reflection) but in this case, it is being in a meditative state with your eyes open, and as the observer without judgment, while in positive self talk to your own reflection.

When I looked into my mirror every day, I affirmed that I was ten years younger biologically. Did it work, yes! This was and is due to the power of belief through affirmation with feeling and acceptance, and then living in that ageless consciousness!

As I gazed into the mirror, I observed my physical facial image as it was, without judgment. I looked deeply into my eyes which reflected back to me (as the observer), the depth of my soul nature. My soul is what I connected with for my transformative work.

I felt and knew that my inner-self was an integral part of the divine Creator, for I Am his child. I personally saw God the Creator, as a vibrating field of pure divine loving intelligence with Infinite possibilities!

I knew then, when I first began to tap into this natural creative energetic field, that I just needed to surrender to all possibilities, including allowing myself to be ageless! In the process I began to reverse my biological age, as I stepped into that consciousness.

In the "Field" I saw myself through the eyes of my soul, as a vibrating source of Light energy, with all of my cells dancing the divine dance of wholeness, youth and vitality! And, the transformation began and it has not stopped to this writing date in 2015. I still am in the "no age" or, ageless expression of consciousness.

When I personally say, I am 82 (or) beyond as the years go by, this chronological age has no power over me, because of my ageless consciousness, and I never affirm this actual chronological age in front the mirror or at any other anytime! When I tell people my age, it is for their learning purpose only, as I have no attachment to my yearly birthdays.

I am convinced the key to transformation is first established in the power of belief. Then, it is allowing oneself to abide in, and to be the consciousness of that belief, which is actually being the active part of that perception!

Of course, living a healthy physical lifestyle is also important for being ageless. This lifestyle also includes emotionally embracing life, and doing ones best to stay out of judgment of "self." It is learning to love yourself unconditionally. Only then, can you refrain from judgment of others, which allows you to be more loving and compassionate toward all of life.

When we live in wholeness we create happiness for ourselves and for others! Wholeness is Agelessness!

How to do Mirror work:

You can use a hand mirror or wall mirror, or even a compact sized mirror to do your daily ageless "active meditation" exercise. Mirror work in order to be effective, must be done for 30 days in a row. The number three vibration represents creativity, add the zero, and you have God power! It only takes a few minutes of your daily life for mirror work and the benefits are great!

1. Take 3 deep breaths to center and relax yourself.
2. Casually observe your reflection without judgment.
3. Speak these words: Your name, and then say, "I give myself complete permission to love myself unconditionally, and with this love I claim agelessness". Example: Joy, I give myself complete permission to love myself unconditionally, and with this love I claim agelessness!
4. Look yourself deeply in the eyes, (the windows to your soul).
5. Observe what your eyes are reflecting back to you as a silent message.
6. Relax into your soul "inner being" with complete trust.
7. Your soul is non-judgmental.
8. Stay connected with your eyes.
9. Affirm and feel the sense of being ageless with the statement of: "I AM" now filled with the consciousness of youth and vitality. I Am Ageless Now!

*When you truly feel you have connected with agelessness, you can name your new biological age (within reason), perhaps ten years younger, while looking into the mirror and saying your name first, and then your new age. I like to say thank you, for being in gratitude is powerful for the manifestation of our desires.

With affirmation, belief and gratitude, you begin to live in a more vital state of consciousness! When you live in "agelessness consciousness," you will act ten years younger, and through the action, you are it!

So, you may be wondering if I am ageless, why assign an age number to myself? You need a goal or a point of reference to act from, in the transformative process of being ageless. From then on, you just forget your new biological age. You do not even give aging a thought! You live and move consistently from the central point of power within yourself. And, as the years go by, you still retain the aspects of agelessness.

Being ageless, is feeling and maintaining a sense of well being and wholeness. Wholeness is living life positively and fully awake, which is a state of awareness. When you are fully awake you are tapping into the Universal Consciousness, which is the natural divine power that is always acting for you, and never against you!

*Because of individual spiritual beliefs and semantics, you may choose to call this divine power any name you wish to assign to it. A label does not change the source, it just is.

Scientific Brain Studies:

Neuro-Science studies show that through brain imagery

studies, the process of inner self reflection, and self talk and mirror work reflection, actually stimulates the prefrontal brain lobes, which causes the brain to switch to a position of creative response and acceptance. The prefrontal lobe response interrupts any negative input from the amygdala brain response that can induce negative thought patterns. If you are interested you can do further research on this data.

Mirror Images:

Mirror image response goes way back to the fairly tale of Snow White. Of course the wicked witch used the mirror in a narcissistic way, by saying "Mirror, Mirror on the wall, who is the most beautiful of all!" And you know where that got her!

Ponds and pools of water have always revealed our reflections. Reflections give us self awareness and deep positive messages on all levels, when we know how to apply the work positively for transformation!

The negative is depicted by the Greek Myth Narcissus (narcissism) as represented by a handsome Greek youth, who fell in love with his own reflection in a pond of water. The story goes that he lay gazing by the pool hour after hour... and finally changed into a flower that bears his name, the Narcissus. Well...that was transformation of sorts!

Giving ourselves permission to love ourselves unconditionally is not being Narcissistic. It is an acknowledgement of "higher love" working through our heart, so we can love others more unconditionally as well.

97

If we do not love and appreciate ourselves in a healthy way, it is impossible to truly love others for who they are, and as they are.

So, pick up your mirror and start your ageless work today!

Step 15

How Colors
Can Enhance Your Life

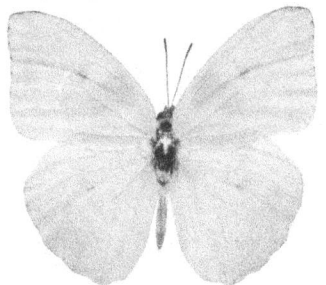

How Colors Effect Us and
How You Can Use Them to Enhance Your Life

Color is the energy of light.

When you see a rainbow in the sky, doesn't it make you feel happy as you gaze at the seven glorious colors?

A rainbow is an optical and metrological phenomenon that causes a spectrum of light to appear in the sky, when the Sun shines onto droplets of moisture or tiny ice crystals in the earths' atmosphere. This takes the form of a multicolored arch of seven colors, with red on the outer part of the arch and violet on the inner section.

Isaac Newton gave us the understanding about light and color. White light is a mixture of colored light. The different colors correspond to light with different wavelengths and are refracted to differing degrees. The separation of colors is known as dispersion. Once the colors in the sunlight are separated by refraction, we are able to distinguish them in the seven colors of the rainbow.

When clear crystals are held up to the sunlight, or if the sun is caught by a crystal hanging in a window, the multifaceted cut crystal will separate the white light and spread rainbow colors on the walls of the room. I love to see nature in action. I have crystals hanging in my sunroom windows.

How do we perceive color? The amazing fast work of judging color begins in the retina, which has three layers of cells. On a broader scale of information...to get past many scientific details...comparisons of neighboring portions of an image leads to our ability to see colors. And we need light to see color. There are precise paths of neural brain messages that also make it possible for us to see the wealth of color, and to distinguish the various shades or hues.

Every frequency of light (color), affects each one of us. Knowing how color affects life itself, you can use color to enhance your personal life experience. Color can help to bring balance and healing to the physical, mental, emotional and spiritual levels of your being!

I have used color therapy on myself and on my Reflexology clients. I have used rainbow lights and swatches of rainbow colors. They give wonderful boosts of energy to the viewer, or promote the feeling of peace and restfulness. It depends on the color being presented.

In the year of 1878, Dr. Edwin Babbit (a medical doctor) published his book entitled The Principals of Light and Color.

His book brought many raised eyebrows form the medical profession! However, his book was the most believable and notable work on light and color of its time.

In Dr. Babbits' medical practice, he incorporated the utilization of different devices that combined rainbow colored filters with both natural and electrical light. With his method of applying light and color to certain body parts of a patient, it was reported that when a selected color was shown directly upon the physical body (on the part that needed healing), health reoccurred in the area that had been sick! He understood the condition that caused the imbalance in the body in the first place, and secondly he knew which color would restore the body to balance.

His many successes of working with light and color were never truly recognized by the medical profession, but they did create enough recognition in the minds of many, so that light and color therapy is still used today by some very valid practitioners.

When applied with knowledge, the following colors will assist you in your pursuit of wellness and agelessness!

Red

When you look at the color of red it stimulates you! It is not a color that you would want to put in your bedroom because it doesn't suggest restfulness.

Red is the color of blood and life energy. It is a life-giving, stimulating force. Physical activity and the energy behind movement are red in vibration. Red is associated with heat. Sexual activity and the creative life force are also imbued with red energy. Many male leaders wear red ties to be noticed, and it makes them feel powerful. Women who wear red dresses are thought to be seductive because they want to be noticed. So, if you want to be known as bold, dynamic or sexy wear red! When you see a red sports car, how does that make you feel? Police are always watching for excess speed in a red car. The expression; "seeing red" alludes to anger. Anger is overheated emotional energy in its negative form. Red is also known as a romantic color as it is associated with Valentine's Day.

How can you enhance your moods and health with red?

You can increase your energy level and your feeling of enthusiasm by exposing yourself to red. When you are feeling tired, wear something red or introduce red into your environment when you need it. If you are feeling fearful or insecure, this hot color will make you feel more confident and bold. Red is a survival color, and can assist you in goal planning and making your dreams come true. Eating red foods, will give your energy level a boost.

Orange

Orange is a warm color. It is a mixture of red and yellow. Orange warms, red burns, and yellow is bright and sunny. Orange gives us the feeling of wanting to move into play and exploration. Orange seems to stimulate movement and to get us involved in projects and life. Orange enhances our thought processes and our curiosity.

How can you enhance your moods and health with orange?

Put orange into your life, for creating a feeling of being interested in life. If you feel nothing exciting is happening and you are bored, get orange! If you are feeling overly responsible and taking yourself too seriously, add orange to your environment.

If you are one who hangs onto the past and can't seem to move forward, this warm color will help you let go. Vibrant orange will help you be more creative, and you will find life is more fun.

Think of orange as recharging you. This lovely vibrant color will also soothe jangled nerves, by helping reduce stress levels. Adding more orange foods will give you more zest for life!

Yellow

Yellow is a happy color. It is bright and warm and makes us think of sunshine. We get a sense of joy and vitality when we see clear bright or soft yellow. Yellow stimulates a feeling of alertness, and enhances the brain-mind functions. It helps us in making decisions. It brightens our outlook on life and can help depression. When you are happy your immune system gets a boost!

How can you enhance your moods and health with yellow?

Adding yellow in your life will lift your spirits. Since it increases the brain-mind functions, you will be able to make clear decisions. Learning abilities are also greatly improved. If you need to learn something, or are doing research, put something yellow near you. If you are forgetful, or know some one that is, introduce more yellow into the environment. Your nervous system will be enlivened with yellow so that you will not experience depression. I add yellow color to my environment in the wintertime, as I live in the dark and cold Northwest.

Adding more yellow food to your diet will be helpful to your digestive system such as golden yellow honey. Honey, boosts your immune system! Eat yellow apples, yellow squash, lemons, grapefruit, and bananas.

Green

Green is for growth and balance. In growth, there is order for expansion. Green can lead us into discovering new paths in life. Green is also related to abundance and to healing.

How can you enhance your moods and health with green?

Use green when you need to break out of confinement of any kind. Allow change to happen naturally. Green will help bring more balance into your life. If you are rigid about certain things, green is a must. Color your life with green for a sense of freedom. Green food is filled with cleansing properties, provides energy, and enhances cellular healing.

Blue

Blue is a restful color and is wonderful for meditation. It is a good color for your bedroom if you have trouble sleeping. It is the color for a peaceful environment. The blue sky and the blue ocean impart a feeling of deep relaxation along with a sense of vastness into areas of never ending expansion.

How can you enhance your moods and health with blue?

Since blue assists with the feeling of peace, it will help you to communicate your ideas and feelings in a relaxed way. Blue encourages compassion and understanding. Use blue to relax you when your emotions have been agitated. Blue is great color for stress management. If you have trouble with insomnia visualize blue, as you tell yourself that you are going to fall asleep quickly, and that you will sleep the entire night, and awaken feeling rested. There are no sky blue colored foods.

Indigo

This dark blue color is mysterious to the beholder. It can deepen your thoughts into introspection. It is associated with the deep blue of the night sky.

How can you enhance your mood and health with indigo blue?

Indigo can take you deep into the mysteries of the spiritual life. It can give you sudden inspiration. It is a key color for seeking deep spiritual connections with God. Indigo is good for enhancing your intuition. Deep blue foods such as dark blue berries dark blue plums and grapes are rich in antioxidants. These indigo foods are good for boosting brainpower.

Violet

Violet is a combination of blue and red. It is interesting that the beginning color of the spectrum is red and that blue is the final mix that creates violet, which brings a circle of completion. Violet is a high vibrating color that merges back into the white light. Beyond violet, our physical eyes no longer detect variant hues of color. Violet increases the imagination, suggesting there may be more colors beyond what our physical eyes can see.

How can you enhance your mood and health with violet?

Put more violet into your environment when you want to heal on the physical level and emotional level, and experience the creative flow of healing spiritual energy in your cells. This color can be helpful in the integration of your physical, mental, emotional, and spiritual well being. It is used in many spiritual and religious ceremonies. It is the color of royalty. It can increase your spiritual connection to the unseen or heavenly worlds. It is a beautiful color to have near you in prayer and meditation. Violet foods are not very prevalent; eggplant is one of the few that I can recall.

White

White is the complete wholeness that contains all the colors. It is the white light.

White is associated with purity. Virgin brides always

wore white. Nowadays, any bride can wear it, virgin or not. White can lead to a new beginning.

How can you enhance your mood and health with white?

White can give a feeling of spaciousness and of purity. New beginnings and new ideas can be generated in white. Visualizing white for cleanliness and purity can fight infection. It is easy to feel a sense of lightness and freedom from all that is holding you back, when white is introduced into the environment.

Black

Black absorbs light. Black conceals and constricts. Black represents the unknown, the mysterious and it often represents that which is hidden in the dark. Black can elicit fear, and thoughts of evil lurking somewhere in the night. Black is mysterious and it is used for funeral attire. Black represents an ending. It is empty space. Black takes you into the void of nothingness.

How can you enhance your mood and health with black?

A dark or black room without light can take you into the void for deep, restful sleep.

Black and white are total opposites. The light of day fades away for the dark of night. All of life is built on opposites: positive and negative, light and dark.

Visualize color for bringing balance into your body and life.

Visualization and thought are very powerful when used together. I have used color visualization in some of my meditations when I needed a certain color for my physical well-being, and also to lift my spirits when I felt a little gloomy. I have found color to be very helpful. Often, I will have a swatch of color to look at first, in order to make my imaging easier to project onto my inner screen of awareness.

If you want to use color to add to your youth and wellness regimen, imagine the color of your choice, to be all around you in the air so it will be easily accessible. Then, allow the color to pervade you entire body by focusing it front of your minds eye. The next step is to breathe it in, and to focus the color into your pineal gland, and into your heart after you feel the color has traveled throughout your entire being.

Sometimes, I form the color I am using into the shape of a flower in my minds eye. Flowers, like the color spectrum are very high in vibration, and are nourishing to the soul, and to the physical self. Every flower is exquisitely beautiful in its color and shape, and each one is unique unto itself. To me, flowers are a reflection of the beauty and love of heaven itself!

The fragrances of flowers are a delight to the senses, and actually carry soothing, healing powers in their essences and colors. Flowers stir our emotions (as does color), as flowers seem to compliment our higher appreciation of life itself. I feel that flowers and colors are gifts to be treasured, and help us to rediscover the beautiful and colorful fragrance of life, that is the very essence of our soul. This is why I suggest you learn to visualize color and flowers together from time to time.

If you cannot visualize color and form in your mind, just THINK it, and look at the color beforehand, and at a flower, or picture of a flower, if you intend to use both. "Thoughts are things on airy wings," and carry power.

Step 16

Health and Beauty of Your Skin

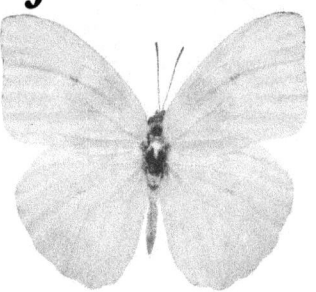

Natural Lotions and Potions

Your skin is the largest organ of your body and reflects your overall health condition.

Try to aim for toxic free living as best you can because, your skin absorbs everything you put on it, and that product is carried into your blood stream in minutes!

I want to offer a word of caution for those of you who may use the facial product Botox®.

Think about what Botox® is before you use it. Botox® is Botulism, a poison. However, it has been approved by the FDA for cosmetic use for treating lines and wrinkles on the face. Thousands of women opt to have this cosmetic procedure done about every four to five months, so their face will look stress free, lineless, and younger. Most experience minimum side effects, if any, but there have been exceptions. Do your own research and then make up your mind. Personally, I will never use Botox® as the skin is an organ, and the product will most likely enter the blood stream to some extent. Skin patches are used for estrogen treatments, birth control and to subdue the desire to smoke, because the treatment product does not remain locked onto the skin, it is absorbed into the body.

We all carry toxins in our body because we now live in a man made toxic world. Some people are over laden with toxins, and it can show as a lack of luster in their skin. Toxins can also cause certain skin problems.

Along with better lifestyle choices, cleansing and care of the skin is vital for the health of the outer layers of your skins tissue. Cleansing with harsh soaps can cause dryness and a lack of luster to your skin. I like to use natural products because they work so well and brighten my skin. Natural skin care products can be found in health food stores and "on line." An added benefit of going natural is the inexpensive prices!

Even though natural beauty products can be purchased for the face, why not get creative and make your own! Here are some beauty recipe ideas for you to try.

Natural Cleansers

Glycerin

This is a gentle cleanser and can be found in bars in most stores. It is one of my favorite cleansers and the bars come with different base scents. It can be used on the face and the body.

Oatmeal and Honey Scrub

Ingredients:

1/2 cup oatmeal

2 Tbsp honey

1 tsp nutmeg

15 drops Lavender Essential Oil

15 drops Tea Tree Oil

Here's how to make it:

Run oatmeal through blender to break up just a little bit. Don't make it powdery, you need texture.

Transfer the Oats into a measuring cup or small bowl.

Add remaining ingredients and stir well. It will be a bit crumbly. If needed, add a bit more honey to get the ingredients to bind together.

Store the mixture in a small plastic or glass container with a lid at room temperature.

One batch should last 2 weeks if used daily.

About the benefits of this scrub:

Oatmeal is excellent for stimulating and exfoliating the skin.

Honey acts as a natural moisturizer, and has healing and soothing properties.

Nutmeg is an astringent, and is anti-bacterial and soothes the skin.

Lavender Oil is ant-inflammatory and soothing.

Tea Tree Oil is an anti-oxidant, an antiseptic, and prevents and heals blemishes.

Natural skin Toners

Apple Cider Vinegar

Would you believe it? Raw, organic bottled Apple Cider Vinegar! The scent goes away when it dries. It is great.

Ingredients:

2 Tbsp. Apple cider vinegar

4 Tbsp. Filtered or distilled water

Store the toner in a small container at room temperature, or you can refrigerate, for a more refreshing feeling. Shake well each time you before use it. Apply with cotton ball. Be careful around delicate eye tissues.

The benefits are:
Balances and restores the skin to natural ph factor.
Evens skin tone.
Dissolves dead skin cells
Tightens pores

Witch Hazel and Rose Water

Ingredients:
¼ cup alcohol free witch hazel
¼ cup filtered water
10 drops of essential rose oil (this can be pricy, but there are brands that are not, shop around).
Always shake before using and store at room temperature.
Benefits:
Brightens skin and closes pores. Rose oil soothes and balances the facial skin, and gives a lovely lingering fragrance.

Sweet Citrus Toner

Ingredients:
½ cup witch hazel
10 drops sweet orange essential oil
Put in container and shake well before each use.
Benefits:
Tones and tightens pores, refreshes. Great for summer!
Brightens skin

Green Tea Toner

1 cup brewed tea
Cool and store in refrigerator
Benefits:

Soothes' irritated skin.

Rose Water

Rose Water or Floral water- for a fragrant facial spray.

Place rose petals, or fragrant flowers, with stems and leaves removed in a bowl. Cover with hot water and let sit overnight.

Strain the next day. Store in a small spray bottle and refrigerate between using.

Benefits:

Refreshes and naturally scents your face and neck on those hot summer days.

Natural Facial Moisturizer

Organic Coconut oil with vitamin E

Ingredients:

½ cup Coconut oil

One teaspoon liquid Vitamin E Oil (for external use)

Seven drops of essential Lavender oil

How to make:

Combine all oils in small bowl and stir well, and that's it! Store the oils in small container with a lid. Keep at room temperature. In cold weather the coconut oil becomes solid, and in the warm weather it can liquefy. Run container under hot water if oil is too solid. Remember a little bit goes a long way. Dip finger tips in the moisturizer and smooth over face with light massage. Dab with a cotton ball if you feel you have too much on.

Benefits:

This moisturizer has many benefits! It is inexpensive and hydrates well. It also creates a protective film that helps to keep out environmental impurities. This combination softens the skin and reduces the appearance of fine lines. A lot of women just use the coconut oil alone. I suggest this is not enough protection. Vitamin E is essential to the total health of your skin. Vitamin E helps to fight signs of aging, as it slows down and refines fine lines. It is an anti-oxidant, and helps to protect the skin from being sun damaged. It also reduces the possibilities of skin cancer. So be certain to add Vitamin E oil to the coconut oil! The Lavender is soothing and gives a lovely finishing scent.

Skin types oily, or dry or balanced, benefit from this naturally created moisturizer, and you get to make sure it is all organic based!

Use the oils in the morning, be sparing, and again at night after cleansing your face.

Note: *I always use glycerin for cleansing my skin in the morning and night. It is mild, gentle and takes all makeup off easily! Glycerin comes in liquid or solid cake forms. It is not a regular soap. As a bonus it is inexpensive!*

Natural Facial Mask

Grapefruit/Egg Facial Mask (Once a week)
Ingredients:

One egg (separated as you will only use the egg white at first). Keep the yoke.

One teaspoon of grapefruit juice

How to make

Beat egg white until fluffy. Next, blend in 1 teaspoon of slightly beaten yoke. Add one teaspoon of the grapefruit juice to the mixture. Blend together, using a spoon.

Apply liberally and evenly to your face, and then lean back and rest for 10 minutes. You may wish to add a thin slice of fresh cucumber over your eye lids to refresh your eyes and skin around the eyes, while the mask is doing its beauty and health work! Afterward, wash with cool water and pat dry. Now use your homemade toner and moisturizer!

Benefits:

Tightens and lifts and brightens your face. Your face is also bathed in natural minerals.

Body Lotion

Coconut oil with Shea Butter

Ingredients:

4.5 oz of Shea Butter

¼ cup of raw organic Coconut oil

3 Tbsp Jojoba Oil

1 Tbsp Calendula Oil

How to make

Mix all ingredients (using a heavy spoon) together in a bowl, finish with electric or hand held egg beater to blend well. Fill small glass jars with the lotion. Refrigerate left over Shea Butter, to keep the Butter fresh, so you can make more lotion at a later time. Keep Lotion you want to use at room temperature. You should have enough for 2 months from this recipe.

Benefits:

Benefits are having a soft, moisturized and weather protected skin. This lotion is especially good for overly dry skin, but works for all skin types.

Note: The facial coconut oil with the Vitamin E recipe can also be used on especially dry skin areas on the body.

Enjoy your creativity and beautiful, healthy skin!

Note: *Why spend hundreds of dollars on expensive skin care products when you can be your own chemist? Check out the internet for even more lotion and potion ideas.*

A bit of Lotion and Potion history from ancient civilizations:

The earliest use of moisturizers and other skin concoctions dates back to the Mesolithic era 10,000 years ago!

Depending upon the region, women of Pre-Columbus era in Latin America used avocado oil, while in Brazil an Africa palm oil was used for skin care. Others, like the Native Americans used animal fats to soften and insulate their skin. The ancient Greeks used olive oil. The Bible even states that olive oil and spices were used for lotions.

The Sumerians created emollients from pulverized plant and animal material, and combined them with wine and tree oils, before applying to their bodies.

Ancient Egypt's Cleopatra was famous for her oils, lotions and make up. For her skin treatments, it is recorded that she took milk baths to keep her skin soft and ageless. Milk and citrus fruit contains natural AHA, which is "Alpha Hydroxy Acid". AHA is great for exfoliating the skin, and minimizing fine lines in the face. This ingredient can be found in many of today's beauty products, as it helps to gently eliminate dead skin cells.

Cleopatra used olive oil and sesame oil for moisturizing and softening her skin. She also used honey for facials and skin care.

About Honey

Honey can be used as a facial mask. It must be raw honey. It can clear and smooth the skin on the face. Honey is a natural humectant, which means it attracts and holds in moisture keeping the skin well hydrated. If you want to try a honey facial treatment, apply a thin coat of honey avoiding the skin directly under the eyes. After 5 minutes you can rinse it off. Your skin will retain the moisture from the water.

I hope you enjoyed learning about how to create your own natural skin care products, and "tidbits" from history!

Step 17

Joy's
Acupressure Face Lift

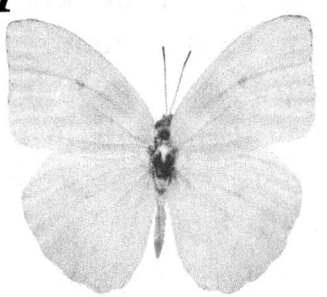

The Natural "Do It Yourself" Acu-Point Facelift

It's never too early or too late to begin something for age reversal and prevention!

Acupressure is an adjunct therapy that you can perform on yourself, that can bring forth a more youthful appearance.

Acupressure Face Lift, which I have coined as "Acu-Point," stimulates the muscles and the skin by triggering key acupressure points that release vital energy into the face. This technique when used as a regular weekly practice will bring forth a vibrant appearance and a gentle, but noticeable face lift. It also softens the lines in the face.

It is suggested that you apply acupressure to your face daily for seven days. After the seven days, once a week should be your routine. You may begin to notice changes in your skin in about six to eight weeks. This method of application must be continued on a regular once a week basis for lasting results.

What is Accupressure?

Acupressure is Acupuncture without needles. It has been widely used in the Orient for well over 5000 years!

It is a proven method that helps to restore the natural balance in body functions, and promotes a sense of youthful vitality and well-being. It is now used in the west as an alternative therapy.

"Acupressure is finger contact with the skin."

When you know exactly where to place your fingers you will be touching certain KEY points that are on the "meridians" or energy channels. These channels are thought to carry the vital life force energy throughout the body systems that restore balance and health.

These channels run through the face as well as the body. When KEY POINTS on the face are stimulated, your own life force energy rushes forth and begins to restore balance.

Balance helps to restore a more youthful appearance, and since the meridians run all through the body, your body will receive benefits as well.

By the time you complete the natural face-lift routine your face should feel stimulated and filled with tingly energy! You may also feel a sense of well being along with the feeling of relaxation.

As a suggestion, a great time to lift your face is while you watch TV. A very relaxing time... is when you are soaking in a bubble bath!

Natural Acu-Point Face Lift

Joy's Way Acu-Point
Beauty and Regeneration Routine

Acu-Point Step 1

These two points (note arrows) open energy to the entire face. Note: The thin muscles in this area of the forehead will be stimulated and relaxed by the finger action of vibrating in an up and down motion for 30 seconds. Then just press and hold using firm pressure for 30 seconds.

You may immediately feel the circulation opening up your face and may experience soothing sensations in other parts of the body.

This *Acu-Point* is located directly in line with the pupils of the eyes. In some cases due to facial structures the points may be a little higher or lower or to the left or right. By a little adjustment of your fingers, you will find the small notch openings.

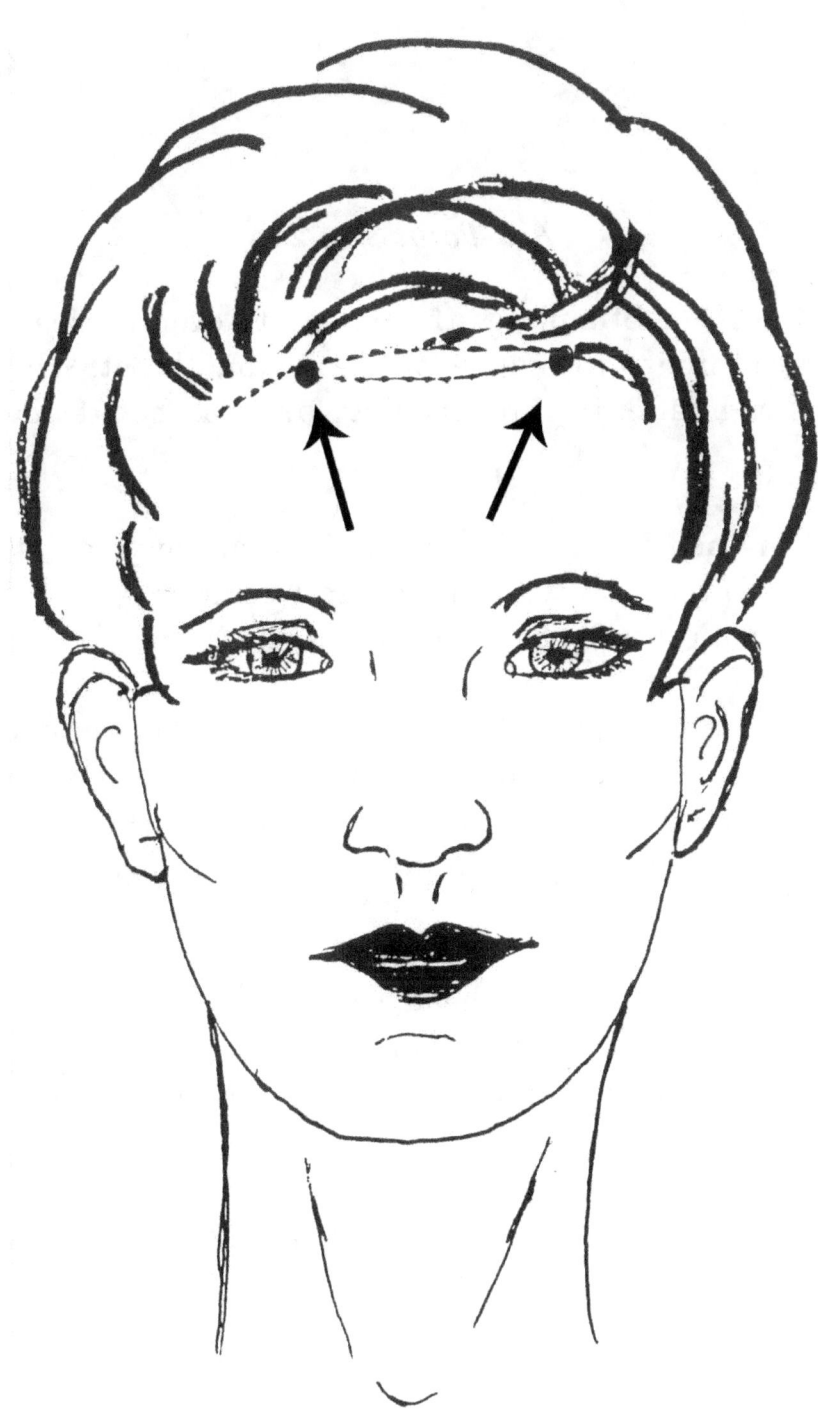

Acu-Point Step 2

Point #1 Stimulates the energy to even a greater degree through the entire facial area and throat. When used right after the first opening points on the previous page.

This point is to be pressed simultaneously on the center of the brow with the soft spot point in the center of the top forward part of the cranium.

This cranial point connection is not to be vibrated. Just press in and hold the 2 points together for about 1/2 a minute then release the soft spot on the skull and vibrate for the next 1/2 minute the point on the center of the forehead only.

Point #2 On the forehead, softens the lines and lifts and tones the brow. These points are to be found directly below the first points that are located in the hairline at brow area.

You may wish to refer back to page one.

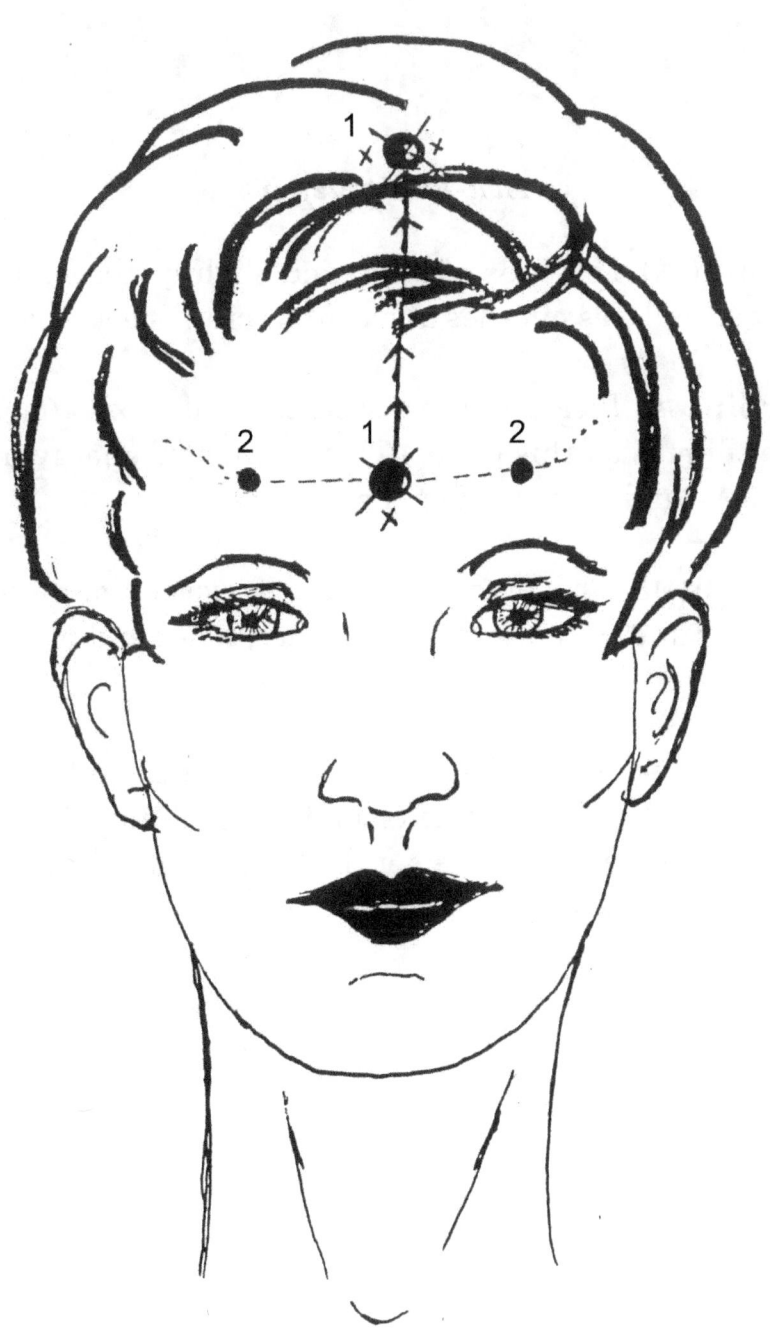

Acu-Point Step 3

Point #1 Far ends of brow and slightly above. This point stimulates muscles and softens crow's feet creases.

Point #2 Inside the eye-sockets right next to nose. (Use thumbs on this point.) This stimulates energy into eye, nose and center of facial areas.

Point #3 The outside corner of eyes. Again, this prevents and softens crow's feet lines, tones and plumps skin around eyes.

Point #4 The ridge of eye-sockets straight down under pupils. This prevents and helps diminish bags under eyes. Improves general skin condition of skin below the eye area.

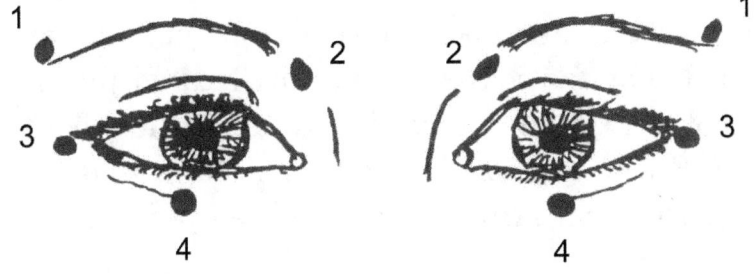

Acu-Point Step 4

Point #1 Small notches are found just upper ridge of eye-socket. They should be located just about center of eye pupil. Press lightly and hold about 1/2 minute. Stimulates energy in upper eye to a gentle lift and improves skin in that part of eye area.

Point #2 Small notches are found just under the lower ridge of eye-socket. Should be located just about center of eye pupil. Press lightly and hold about 1/2 minute. Prevents and helps diminish bags under eyes. Improves general skin condition below eye area.

Point #3 Small depression just below #2 top upper cheekbone area. Press and hold about 1/2 minute. Sends extra energy into lower eye area to strengthen tissue and muscle under the eyes and upper cheek areas.

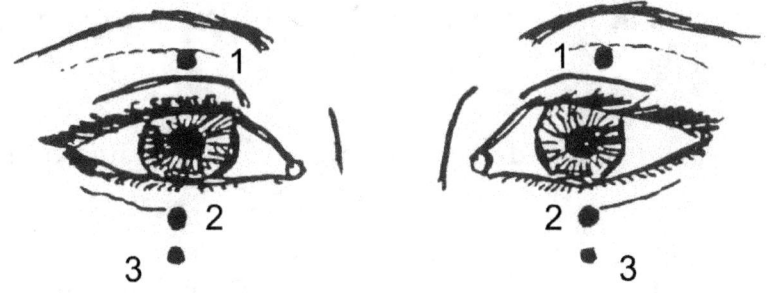

Acu-Point Step 5

Point #1 This point is located outside corner of eyes, feel for elongated openings

Point #2 Lower ridge of eye...more eye energy is released to soften lines and improve skin condition around eye area, you will find small notches in the eye socket ridge.

Point #3 Located in center of temples and just behind temples

For all three points use direct contact with medium light touch and press and hold all points about 1/2 minute. All these points soften crow's feet and diminish bags under eyes, by increasing circulation and energy into these delicate areas.

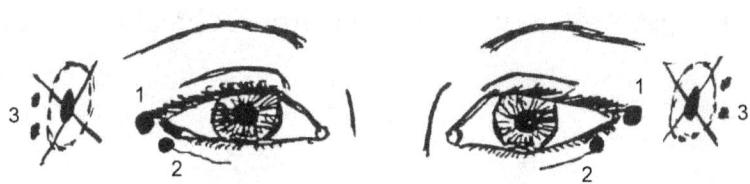

Acu-Point Step 6

Point #1 Located straight down in line with eye pupil, on cheek about even with flare of nostrils.

Point #2 Located just under cheekbone (center)

Push and hold each area about 1/2 minute med-firm pressure. These points tone the large cheek muscle and help to restore the natural contour of the cheek area.

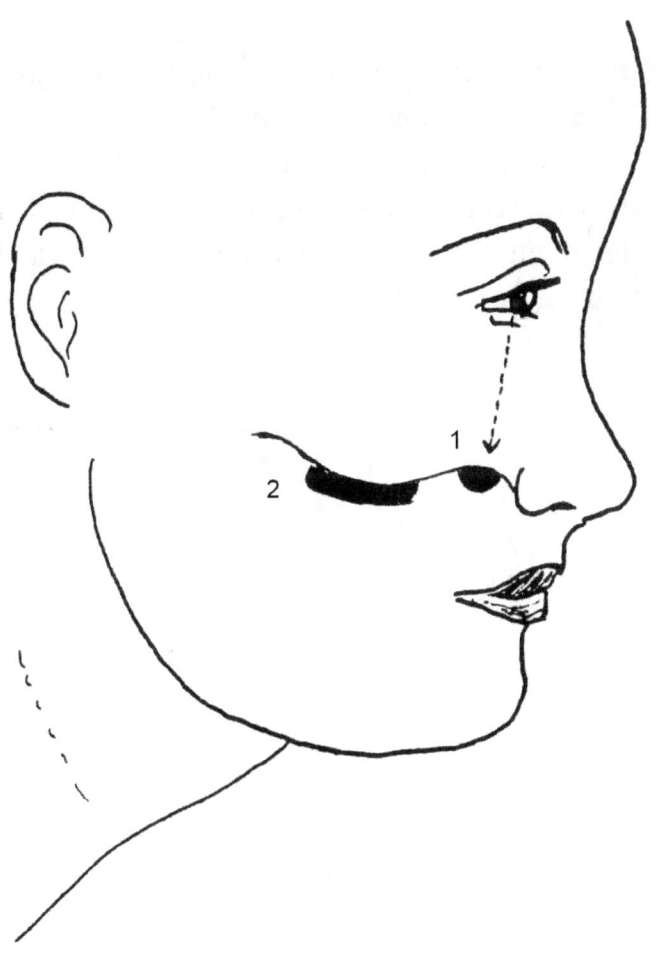

Acu-Point Step 7

Press and hold each point about one minute

Point #1 Located center of cleft above lips. Helpful for vertical lines above the mouth.

Point #2 Midway between lower lip and chin. Softens wrinkles of chin area and stimulates circulation to areas of mouth and entire face.

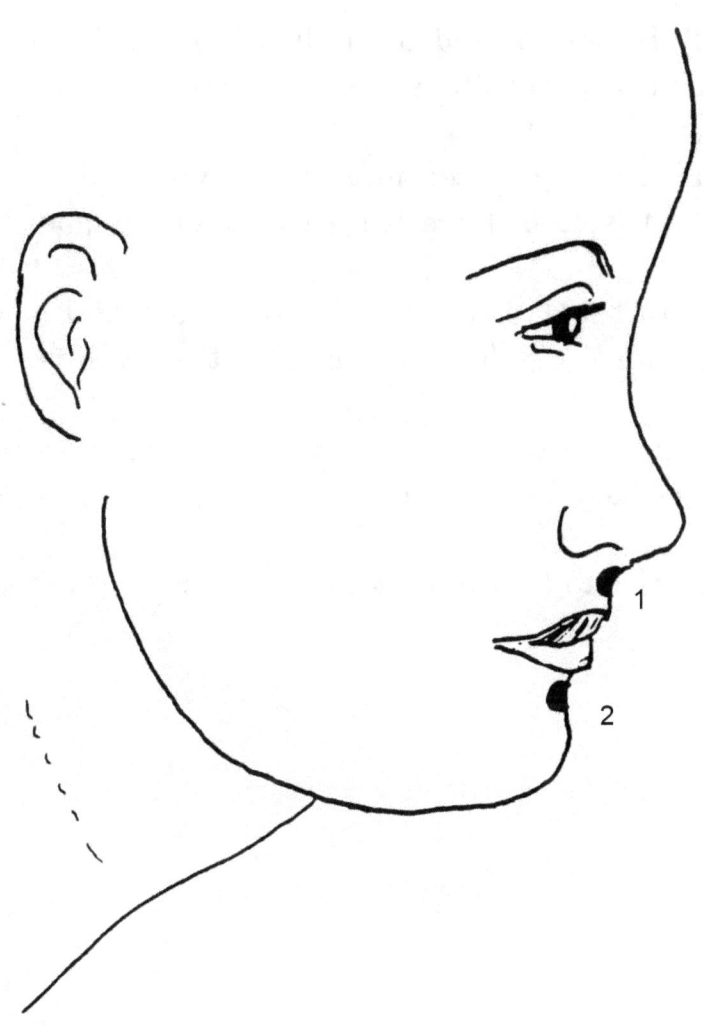

Acu-Point Step 8

Point #1 Located at mid-lip about 1/2" in from corner of mouth. This softens lines at the corner of the mouth.

Point #2 Located midway between chin and lower lip. This softens lines at the corner of the mouth.

Point #3 Lower jaw directly under end of lip line. Small openings. This strengthens the jaw line.

Point #4 Lower Chin centered on the jaw line. This strengthens the jaw line.

Note: Hold all points at least 1/2 minute, medium-firm pressure

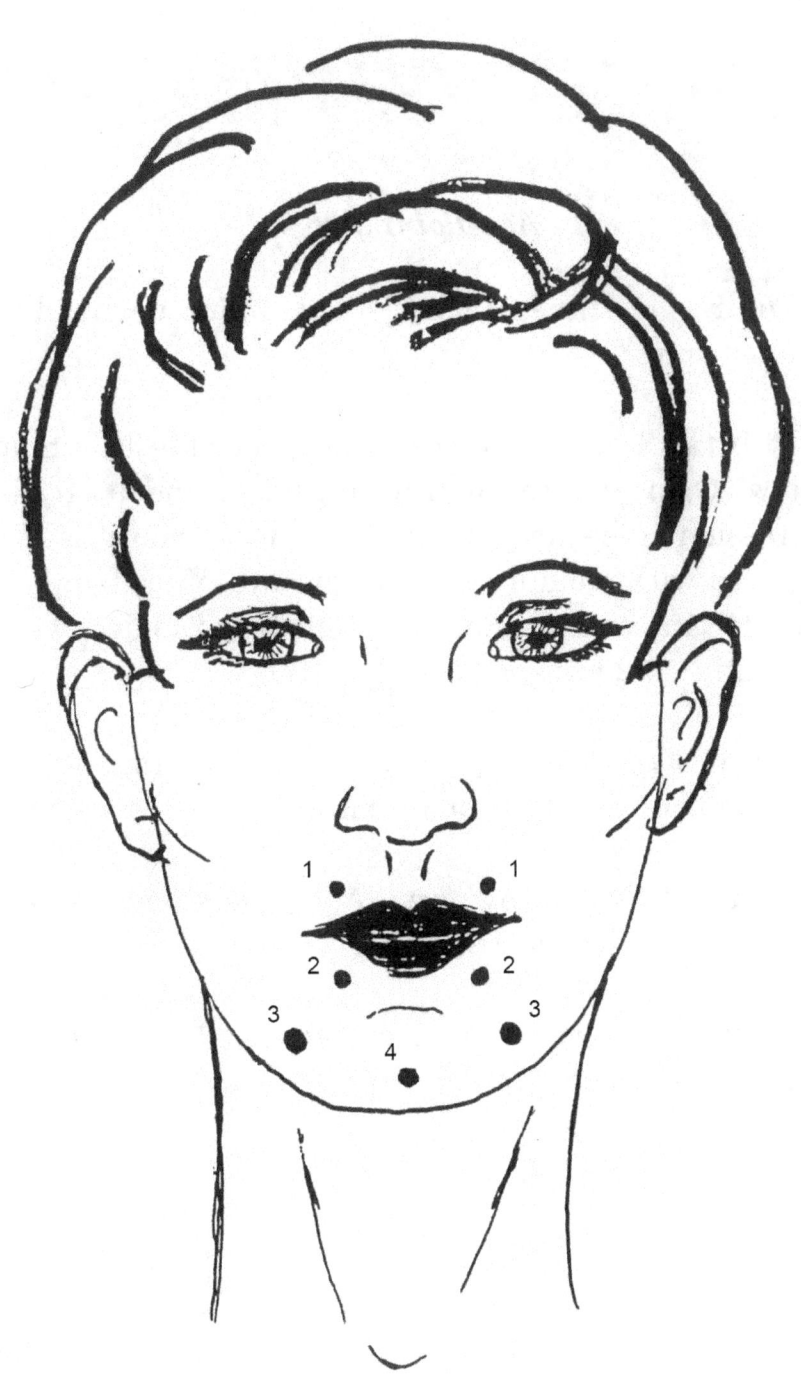

Acu-Point Step 9

To firm Jaw line use these key points, use medium firm pressure

Point #1 Lower Jaw located on large muscle at hinge of jaw. Open mouth slightly until you find it. It is a depression in the jaw. Then close mouth as you stimulate this area with medium to firm pressure. Vibrate up and down for 1/2 minute and then circle toward back of ears for another 1/2 minute.

Point #2 Located just below and in front of ear: Medium firm pressure for 1/2 min.

Point #3 Lower jaw area. Apply medium pressure. Touch and go for a few seconds.

Point #4 Lower chin line notches. Press and hold each for 30 seconds.

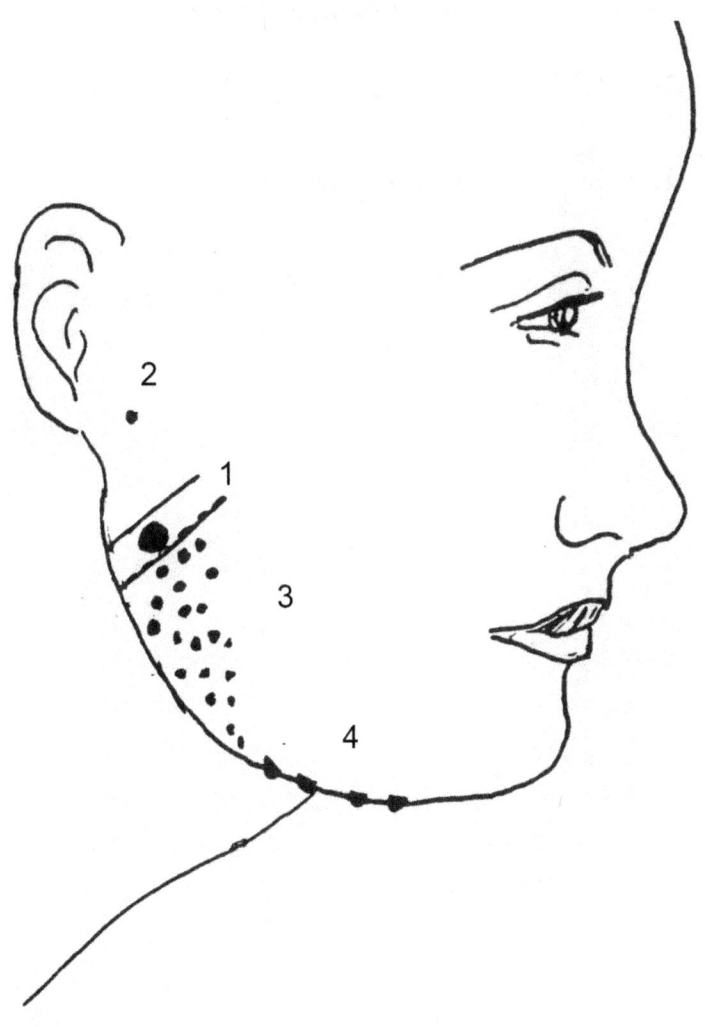

Acu-Point Step 10

Point #1 For throat, vibrate one minute.

Point #2 Press & hold for one minute.

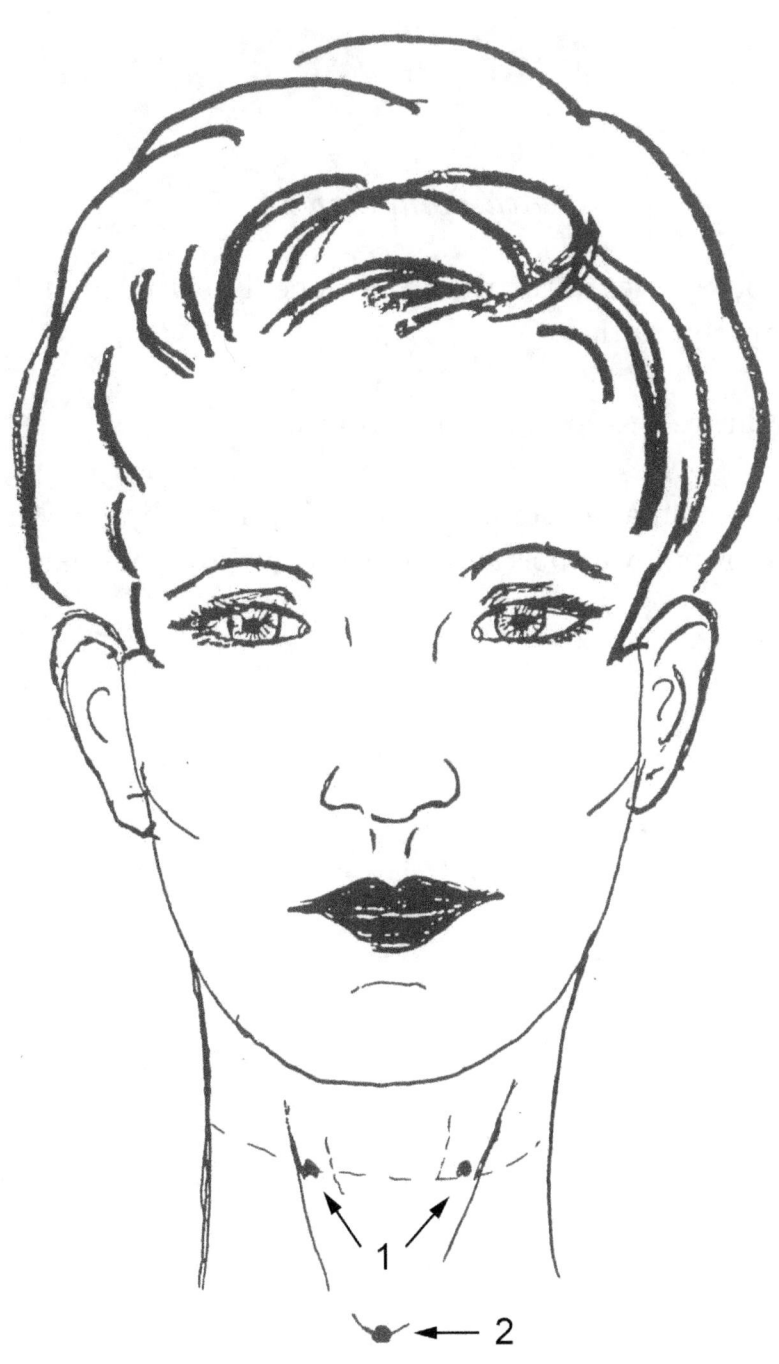

Acu-Point Step 11

Note: Lower dark area on ear lobe. It is used for entire facial stimulation.

Vibrate this area for one minute.

These smaller points can be stimulated by pinching; move from lower portion of ear upward to inner ear.

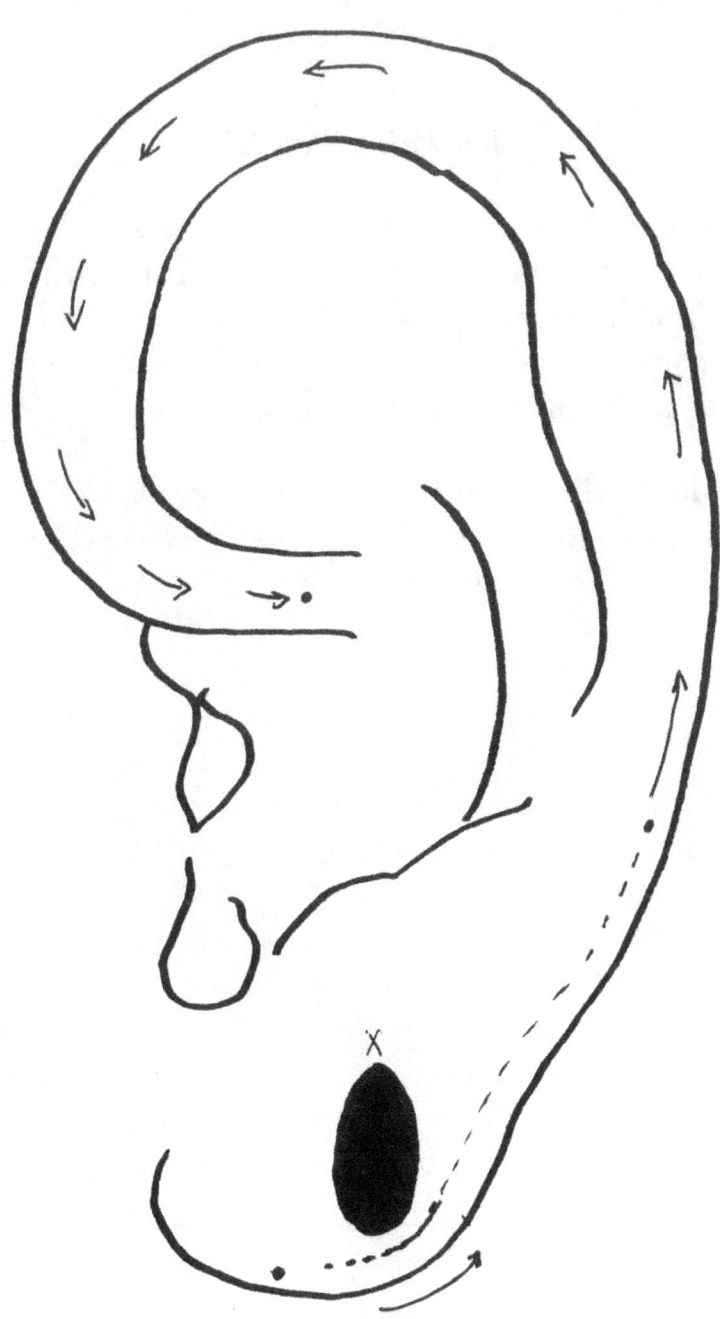

Acu-Point Step 12

Point #1 This is located in the webbed area between the thumb and index finger where they meet in the palm area of the hand only topside. Push and hold on minute leaning pressure toward index finger for energy into face and head. Use medium to firm pressure.

Point #2 Pressure point is the top part of thumb underneath and on top. This represents the facial area. Massage medium pressure for one minute.

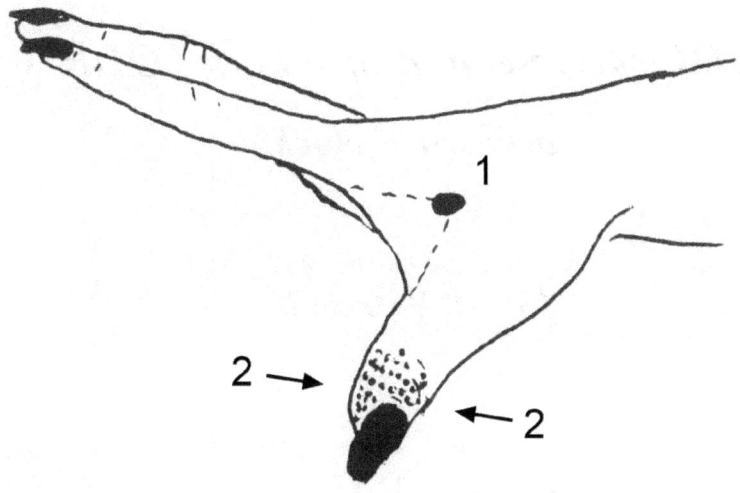

Now YOU have the steps to creating an

Ageless and Healthier YOU!

And

YOU can reset and turn back YOUR

biological clock!

I wish you well!

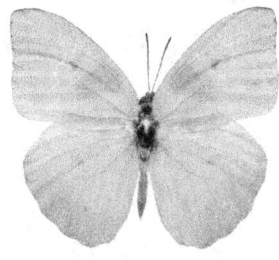

*Joy McMahon is available to speak to your
group or organization.*

*If you wish to contact her go to:
www.joymcmahon.com
or
empressjoy3@yahoo.com*